T0227002

Current Concepts in Cardiovascular Pathology

Guest Editor

GAYLE L. WINTERS, MD

SURGICAL PATHOLOGY CLINICS

surgpath.theclinics.com

Consulting Editor
JOHN R. GOLDBLUM, MD

June 2012 • Volume 5 • Number 2

SAUNDERS an imprint of ELSEVIER, Inc.

W.B. SAUNDERS COMPANY
A Division of Elsevier Inc.

1600 John F. Kennedy Boulevard • Suite 1800 • Philadelphia, Pennsylvania 19103-2899

http://www.surgpath.theclinics.com

SURGICAL PATHOLOGY CLINICS Volume 5, Number 2
June 2012 ISSN 1875-9181, ISBN-13: 978-1-4557-4930-0

Editor: Joanne Husovski

Surgical Pathology Clinics (ISSN 1875-9181) is published quarterly by Elsevier Inc., 360 Park Avenue South, New York, NY 10010. Months of issue are March, June, September, and December. Business and Editorial Office: Elsevier Inc., 1600 John F. Kennedy Blvd., Ste. 1800, Philadelphia, PA 19103-2899. Accounting and Circulation Offices: Elsevier Inc., 3251 Riverport Lane, Maryland Heights, MO 63043. Periodicals postage paid at New York, NY and at additional mailing offices. Subscription prices are $184.00 per year (US individuals), $212.00 per year (US institutions), $91.00 per year (US students/residents), $230.00 per year (Canadian individuals), $240.00 per year (Canadian Institutions), $230.00 per year (foreign individuals), $240.00 per year (foreign institutions), and $112.00 per year (international & Canadian students/residents). Foreign air speed delivery is included in all *Clinics'* subscription prices. All prices are subject to change without notice. **POSTMASTER:** Send address changes to *Surgical Pathology Clinics*, Elsevier, 3251 Riverport Lane, Maryland Heights, MO 63043. Customer Service: 1-800-654-2452 (US). From outside the United States, call 1-314-447-8871. Fax: 1-314-447-8029. E-mail: JournalsCustomerServiceusa@elsevier.com (for print support) and JournalsOnlineSupport-usa@elsevier.com (for online support).

Reprints. For copies of 100 or more, of articles in this publication, please contact the Commercial Reprints Department, Elsevier Inc., 360 Park Avenue South, New York, NY 10010-1710. Tel. (212) 633-3812; Fax: (212) 462-1935; E-mail: reprints@elsevier.com.

Contributors

CONSULTING EDITOR

JOHN R. GOLDBLUM, MD
Chairman, Department of Anatomic Pathology;
Professor of Pathology, Cleveland Clinics,
Lerner College of Medicine, Cleveland Clinic,
Cleveland, Ohio

GUEST EDITOR

GAYLE L. WINTERS, MD
Cardiovascular Pathologist, Associate
Professor of Pathology, Department of
Pathology, Brigham and Women's Hospital,
Harvard Medical School, Boston,
Massachusetts

AUTHORS

MARC HALUSHKA, MD, PhD
Associate Professor of Pathology,
Department of Pathology, Johns Hopkins
University School of Medicine, Baltimore,
Maryland

DYLAN V. MILLER, MD
Director, Intermountain Central Laboratory,
Director, Immunostains and Electron
Microscopy, Associate Professor,
University of Utah, Salt Lake City, Utah

RICHARD N. MITCHELL, MD, PhD
Professor of Pathology and Health Science
and Technology, Department of Pathology,
Brigham and Women's Hospital/Harvard
Medical School, Boston, Massachusetts

ROBERT F. PADERA, MD, PhD
Assistant Professor of Pathology, Department
of Pathology, Brigham and Women's Hospital,
Harvard Medical School, Boston,
Massachusetts

BARBARA A. SAMPSON, MD, PhD
First Deputy Chief Medical Examiner,
Cardiovascular Pathology Consultant, Office
of the Chief Medical Examiner of the City of
New York, New York, New York

FREDRICK J. SCHOEN, MD, PhD
Department of Pathology, Brigham and
Women's Hospital, Harvard Medical School,
Boston, Massachusetts

MICHAEL A. SEIDMAN, MD, PhD
Clinical Fellow in Cardiovascular Pathology,
Department of Pathology, Brigham and
Women's Hospital/Harvard Medical School,
Boston, Massachusetts

JAMES R. STONE, MD, PhD
Department of Pathology, Massachusetts
General Hospital, Harvard Medical School,
Boston, Massachusetts

PAUL A. VANDERLAAN, MD, PhD
Department of Pathology, Brigham and
Women's Hospital, Harvard Medical School,
Boston, Massachusetts

JOHN P. VEINOT, MD, FRCPC
Chairman and Professor, Pathology and
Laboratory Medicine, Department of Pathology
and Laboratory Medicine, Ottawa Hospital,
University of Ottawa, Ottawa, Ontario,
Canada

GAYLE L. WINTERS, MD
Cardiovascular Pathologist, Associate
Professor of Pathology, Department of
Pathology, Brigham and Women's Hospital,
Harvard Medical School, Boston,
Massachusetts

Contents

Cardiovascular Pathology: A Subspecialty of Surgical Pathology   ix

Gayle L. Winters

Native Cardiac Valve Pathology   327

John P. Veinot

> Anatomy of the native cardiac valves, reasons for surgical excision and examination, and a summary of the gross examination and documentation are presented. Aortic stenosis, aortic valve regurgitation, tricuspid and pulmonary valve pathology, mitral stenosis, and mitral insufficiency are each presented with an overview, focused anatomy, and discussion of pathologic diagnosis by gross examination and histology.

Practical Approach to the Evaluation of Prosthetic Mechanical and Tissue Replacement
Heart Valves   353

Paul A. VanderLaan, Robert F. Padera, and Fredrick J. Schoen

> Mechanical and bioprosthetic substitute heart valves have dramatically improved life expectancy and quality of life in patients with valvular heart disease. Complications of substitute heart valves are a relatively infrequent occurrence, often due to thrombosis, infection, or structural/mechanical failure. It is important to accurately identify and systematically evaluate prosthetic heart valves when encountered as surgical pathology specimens or in the autopsy setting.

Cardiac Transplant Biopsies   371

Gayle L. Winters

> The endomyocardial biopsy remains the gold standard for assessing the status of the transplanted heart. It is the most consistently reliable method for the diagnosis and grading of acute cellular and antibody-mediated rejection. Recognition of specimen artifacts and other biopsy findings such as ischemic injury, Quilty effect, infection, and post-transplant lymphoproliferative disorder is important for accurate biopsy interpretation and differentiation from rejection. The endomyocardial biopsy provides important diagnostic information essential for optimal management of cardiac transplant recipients.

Diagnostic Biopsies of the Native Heart   401

James R. Stone

> Endomyocardial biopsy in the nontransplant setting can be diagnostic for particular diseases. Such disorders include amyloidosis, myocarditis, sarcoidosis, iron overload, glycogen storage disorders, and lysosomal storage disorders. The diagnostic features of these disorders on endomyocardial biopsy will be discussed along with the impact of endomyocardial biopsy-based diagnoses on patient management and prognosis.

Pathology of the Aorta   417

Marc Halushka

> The aorta is a distinctive surgical pathology specimen removed most frequently for aneurysm or dissection. Genetic syndromes, inflammatory processes and acquired

diseases of aging result in aortic pathology; these are presented in terms of pathology, differential diagnosis and classification schemes. The pathologic context of a variety of commonly encountered histopathologies is described.

Surgical Pathology of Small- and Medium-Sized Vessels   435

Michael A. Seidman and Richard N. Mitchell

Surgical pathologists encounter blood vessels in virtually every specimen they receive, but pathologies intrinsic to the vessels themselves are distinctly less common. Nevertheless, there are a variety of specific diagnoses and procedures involving vascular specimens that merit the attention of the anatomic pathologist. Etiologically, such pathologies can be broadly grouped into traumatic, degenerative, congenital, inflammatory, infectious, and neoplastic lesions. Major examples of most of these are discussed, including anuerysms, vasculitis, thrombosis/embolism, and atherosclerosis.

Cardiac Tumors   453

Dylan V. Miller

Cardiac neoplasms and other mass-forming lesions are not commonly encountered in surgical pathology practice. Fortunately, for the most part, these fall into a small group of well characterized and readily-recognized entities, although they are not without diagnostic dilemmas. A brief and practical synopsis of cardiac tumors is presented in this section with attention to more frequently encountered and clinically significant diagnostic challenges as well as pertinent clinical associations and prognostic information.

Examination of the Cardiac Explant   485

Barbara A. Sampson

Examination of cardiac explants is a challenge to the surgical pathologist. This is due to the complex anatomy of the heart, the numerous pathologies unique to the heart, and the complexities of cardiovascular interventions including the transplant procedure itself. The dissection technique described permits complete evaluation of the heart with good photographic and histologic documentation while maintaining the integrity of the specimen.

Pathologic Evaluation of Cardiovascular Medical Devices   497

Robert F. Padera

Cardiovascular devices such as coronary artery stents, ventricular assist devices, pacemakers, automated implantable cardioverter-defibrillators and septal closure devices are life saving and improve quality of life for millions of patients each year. Complications of these devices include thrombosis/thromboembolism, infection, structural failure and adverse material-tissue interactions. These findings should be sought when these devices are encountered on the surgical pathology bench or at autopsy.

Index   523

SURGICAL PATHOLOGY CLINICS

FORTHCOMING ISSUES

**Current Concepts in Breast Pathology:
Diagnostic Dilemmas and New Insights**
Stuart Schnitt, MD, and Sandra Shin, MD,
Guest Editors

Current Concepts in Molecular Pathology
Jennifer Hunt, MD, *Guest Editor*

Current Concepts in Placental Pathology
Rebecca Baergen, MD, *Guest Editor*

RECENT ISSUES

Current Concepts in Bone Pathology
John D. Reith, MD, *Guest Editor*

Current Concepts in Head & Neck Pathology
Mary S. Richardson, MD, *Guest Editor*

Current Concepts in Soft Tissue Pathology
Elizabeth A. Montgomery, MD, *Guest Editor*

**Current Concepts in Surgical Pathology
of the Pancreas**
N. Volkan Adsay, MD, and Olca Basturk, MD,
Guest Editors

RELATED INTEREST

Heart Failure Clinics, July 2011 (Vol. 7, No. 3)
Cardio-oncology Related to Heart Failure
Daniel J. Lenihan, MD, and Douglas B. Sawyer, MD, PhD, *Guest Editors*

**DOWNLOAD
Free App!**

Review Articles
THE CLINICS

NOW AVAILABLE FOR YOUR iPhone and iPad

Cardiovascular Pathology: A Subspecialty of Surgical Pathology

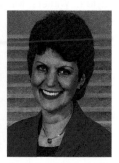

Gayle L. Winters, MD
Guest Editor

For hundreds of years, anatomists, physiologists, and physicians studied the cardiovascular system at autopsy. Cardiovascular pathologists were autopsy pathologists. Within only the last 50 years, the advent of cardiopulmonary bypass, cardiovascular surgical techniques, endomyocardial biopsy, and cardiac transplantation has brought cardiovascular specimens to the surgical pathology bench. These specimens range in size from 0.2 cm (endomyocardial biopsy) to the entire heart (explant). Compared to other areas of surgical pathology, cardiovascular pathology is a "new" subspecialty. I can remember opening a surgical pathology specimen container in 1984 and seeing an entire heart for the first time.

Unfortunately, many surgical pathologists did not embrace the arrival of cardiovascular specimens. Cardiovascular pathology, for the most part, is not tumor pathology. It requires knowledge of cardiac anatomy, cardiac physiology, cardiology, and cardiac surgical procedures. In fact, in some European countries, it is common for cardiovascular pathologists to be trained in clinical cardiology. The increasing importance of making a diagnosis on cardiovascular specimens from living patients put pressure on surgical pathology divisions to find someone to deal with these specimens. Cardiovascular diagnoses could now impact living patients. Additional pressure came during the 1980s from the widely expanding cardiac transplant programs that insisted on cardiac pathology expertise. In more recent years, cardiovascular pathologists have not only had to deal with cardiovascular tissue itself, but with the results of interventional procedures—we must examine stents, pacemakers and defibrillators, prosthetic valves, and ventricular-assist devices. In addition, rapidly growing knowledge in the area of molecular pathology has played an ever-expanding role in how we process tissue and classify cardiovascular diseases.

Cardiovascular pathology is a non-boarded subspecialty of pathology. Although a few cardiovascular pathology fellowships are available, many cardiovascular pathologists practicing today are self-taught. In 1985, cardiovascular pathologists formed the Society for Cardiovascular Pathology (SCVP), which has approximately 200 members worldwide. *Cardiovascular Pathology*, the official journal of the Society, was first published in 1992. The primary goals of SCVP are educational and collegial since many cardiovascular pathologists are the sole person in that specialty within their department. It is important that surgical pathologists recognize their limitations in dealing with cardiovascular specimens, particularly those not commonly encountered, and seek consultation from cardiovascular pathologists with more expertise in the specific area.

In this volume of *Surgical Pathology Clinics* devoted to Cardiovascular Pathology, we attempt to provide useful, practical information on the majority of cardiovascular specimens that may arrive on the surgical bench—valves (native and prosthetic), endomyocardial biopsies (native and transplant), blood vessels ranging from large (aorta) to small, cardiac tumors, and an approach to the explanted heart and cardiovascular devices. In the tradition of this series, each article is replete with photos and has summary boxes

Surgical Pathology 5 (2012) ix–x
doi:10.1016/j.path.2012.04.002

containing key features, differential diagnoses, and pitfalls.

I am indebted to all my coauthors, who have provided their time and expertise. My special thanks to our two cardiac pathology fellows, Michael Seidman and Paul VanderLaan, who have each taken on first authorship of a chapter while performing all of their "routine" duties and preparing for Pathology Boards. Thanks to Dr John Goldblum, Consulting Editor, and Elsevier for remembering to include Cardiovascular Pathology in the *Surgical Pathology Clinics* series and Joanne Husovski of Elsevier for her patience, encouragement, and support.

Gayle L. Winters, MD
Department of Pathology
Brigham and Women's Hospital
Harvard Medical School
75 Francis Street
Boston, MA 02115, USA

E-mail address:
gwinters@partners.org

DEDICATION

This issue is dedicated to my Dad for many years of guidance, encouragement, and support.

NATIVE CARDIAC VALVE PATHOLOGY

John P. Veinot, MD, FRCPC

KEYWORDS

• Endocarditis • Heart • Regurgitation • Stenosis • Valve • Gross examination

ABSTRACT

Anatomy of the native cardiac valves, reasons for surgical excision and examination, and a summary of the gross examination and documentation are presented. Aortic stenosis, aortic valve regurgitation, tricuspid and pulmonary valve pathology, mitral stenosis, and mitral insufficiency are each presented with an overview, focused anatomy, and discussion of pathologic diagnosis by gross examination and histology.

OVERVIEW

Native cardiac valves may be stenotic, insufficient, or involved by infective or non-infective vegetations. Valves that are surgically excised are examined for a number of reasons[1]:

1. To document the surgical indication
2. To correlate pathology with pre-operative diagnosis, hemodynamics, imaging, and suspected complications
3. To document or rule out infective endocarditis
4. To determine the etiology and pathobiology of the valvular lesion which may affect its natural history, surgical risk, post-operative prognosis and association with systemic disease
5. To assess whether another operation could be done on a future similar patient.

Dysfunction of a cardiac valve results from either structural or functional abnormalities of the valve. Valves that are stenotic usually have some structural abnormality-usually fibrosis or calcification. In contrast, regurgitant valves do not always have anatomic abnormalities present with the excised specimen. In regurgitation the abnormality may be related to the valve or to the surrounding supporting structures.

GROSSING AND SECTIONING CONSIDERATIONS FOR NATIVE VALVE EVALUATION

Gross examination and documentation of findings is vital for the evaluation of native valves.[2]

- Valves should be carefully examined for the presence of thrombus or vegetation. If thrombus is noted then sampling for microbiological culture should be considered.
- For cultures, a piece of the thrombus or vegetation is recommended. Swabs are not useful.
- Material can also be submitted for ancillary and molecular studies including electron microscopy,

> ### Key Points
> ### NATIVE CARDIAC VALVE PATHOLOGY
>
> - Careful gross examination is the key to accurate diagnosis of valve disease
>
> - Histologic sectioning may be useful in determining acquired from congenital bicuspid aortic valves and in cases of storage disease and drug related pathology
>
> - All thrombi should be sectioned and stains performed for bacteria and fungi
>
> - Gram stain and silver fungal stain should always be done together
>
> - The cause of valve stenosis is usually apparent from examination of the valve; this is not always the case with regurgitant valves
>
> - In regurgitant valves the cause of the dysfunction may be in adjacent supporting tissues such as the aorta or the ventricle

Department of Pathology and Laboratory Medicine, Ottawa Hospital, University of Ottawa, 501 Smyth Road, CCW Room 4121, Box 117, Ottawa, Ontario K1H 8L6, Canada
E-mail address: jpveinot@toh.on.ca

Surgical Pathology 5 (2012) 327–352
doi:10.1016/j.path.2012.03.001
1875-9181/12/$ – see front matter © 2012 Elsevier Inc. All rights reserved.

immunofluorescence, polymerase chain reaction (PCR) or other molecular techniques.[3–6] Some suggest that PCR may be a better diagnostic tool than culture, especially after anti-microbial therapy, but there remains concern about false positives and background contamination.[5–7]

- Photographs of the inflow and outflow valve surfaces are helpful to document the gross appearance.
- Excised valve cusps or leaflets may be received in their entirety, but sometimes only portions of valves are submitted (especially with valve repair). The dimensions of the specimens should be recorded.
- In atrioventricular valves, the leaflets, commissures, chords, attached papillary muscle, and any annular tissue should be examined for thickening, fusion, irregular edges, defects and calcification.
- Semilunar valves should be examined for the cusp number, presence of a raphe, fusion of commissures, calcification and defects or irregularities including fenestrations and perforations. X-ray is useful to visualize the calcification.
- Submitting tissue in fixative for ultrastructural examination is recommended for storage disease evaluation. All the tissues from the container must be assessed as the valve pieces may be accompanied by pieces of aorta or other cardiac structures.
- Most diagnoses can be made with gross examination and a hematoxylin and eosin (H&E) stained slide.
- Sectioning is still debatable, but the trend is to consider sectioning most valves. All valves with thrombi need to be sectioned to rule out infection. Sections are usually made perpendicular to the line of closure. An H&E stained slide should be generated for each block.

Other optional (not routinely done on every case) stains include:

- Masson trichrome, Azan-Mallory, or Sirius red (to document the degree of fibrosis)
- Verhoeff van Gieson (VVG) elastic stain, Movat pentachrome stain, and/or alcian-PAS stain (to characterize the size and composition of fibrous onlays, the degree of ground substance accumulation, and the degree of underlying native valve destruction).

The elastic stain is probably the most useful of these optional stains. It may also be useful to help determine if a bicuspid aortic valve is an acquired post-inflammatory bicuspid valve or a congenitally bicuspid valve. If one obtains a horizontal section through the raphe or commissure the two "v" shaped pieces may be stained with the elastic stain. Following the elastic layers helps determine whether the area is fused from two cusps or represents a single cusp.[2,8]

A Gram stain should always be accompanied by a silver stain.[6,9] These stains should be done on valves with thrombi and in areas of valve surface erosion. With treatment, Gram-positive bacteria stain variably purple and then Gram negative before losing their Gram staining all together.[10] Silver stains will often still show the bacteria and will detect fungi. Giemsa, Ziehl Neelson/acid-fast bacilli (AFB), and PAS stains are also useful stains in selected cases. In carcinoid syndrome, or drug related pathology immunostains for muscle specific actin (MSA) or smooth muscle actin (SMA) delineate and characterize the fibromuscular plaques.

AORTIC VALVE ANATOMY

Degenerative (age related) change of aortic valves is the most common cause of adult aortic valve stenosis encountered in North America.[11] In age-related degeneration there are 3 cusps that undergo degeneration after decades of normal function:

1. Right
2. Left
3. Posterior or non-coronary cusp.

The non-coronary cusp is usually slightly larger than the other two cusps. Between each cusp and its adjacent cusp there is a commissure which separates them. The cusps have free edges and lines of closure. Near the commissures there are often horizontal cusp defects termed fenestrations, normal structures that become more prominent with age. In the middle of each cusp there is a nodule on the ventricle side along the line of closure termed the nodule of Ariantus. All along the closure line, and especially at the nodule, small whisker like fronds termed Lambl's excrescences may develop.

The annulus of the aortic valve is not a ring but is shaped like a crown or a corona. Each cusp is attached along this fibrous crown leaving intercommissural spaces between the cusps. Just above the aortic valve there is a tapered area with an intimal ridge termed the sinotubular junction. The left and non-coronary cusps of the aortic valve are in fibrous continuity with the anterior mitral leaflet. In disease process such as infective endocarditis, infection can easily spread between the two adjacent valve structures.

The valve cusps are composed of three layers[12]:

1. Fibrosa
2. Ventricularis
3. Spongiosa.

With valve pathology, especially rheumatic disease, these layers may not be easily discernable due to the alterations in valve structure. The fibrosa is the major structural component of the cusp. The spongiosa, the "shock absorber" of the cusp, is composed chiefly of proteoglycans, collagen, fibroblasts, mesenchymal cells and valve interstitial cells. The ventricularis layer contains prominent amounts of elastic fibers and is thickened focally along the line of valve closure forming the nodulus Arantii on the aortic cusps, and the nodulus Morgagni on the pulmonary cusps.

AORTIC STENOSIS OVERVIEW

Stenosis of the aortic valve is usually the result of cusp pathology, commonly fibrosis, calcification and commissural fusion. The most common causes of aortic valve stenosis include[11,13]:

- Calcific degenerative (age related) changes
- Post-inflammatory changes–usually rheumatic
- Congenitally bicuspid valve.

Another, less common cause of valvular aortic stenosis is congenitally unicuspid valve. In general, age related calcific degenerative disease is increasing in incidence, congenital valve disease remains stable at about 1 to 2% of the population and post-inflammatory/rheumatic valve disease is on the decline in North America, but remains a major cause of valve disease in the developing world.

DEGENERATIVE CALCIFIC VALVE STENOSIS

In age-related degeneration the 3 cusps undergo degeneration after decades of normal function. The cusps are separate and the commissures are not fused. The process probably begins with lipid accumulation, but eventually calcium and bone are deposited in an arch like configuration in each cusp (**Fig. 1**A). The top of each arch is directed at the free edge of the cusp with the calcium ridge extending to the base of the side

Fig. 1. (*A*) Gross photograph of a degenerative aortic valve with aortic stenosis. This was removed from an elderly man. There are 3 separate cusps with relatively localized calcium and no commissural fusion. (*B*) Photomicrograph of the aortic valve. Although considered in the past to be degenerative and passive, microscopy demonstrates an active process with calcification (C) and inflammatory (I) cells (hematoxylin phloxine saffron, x 200).

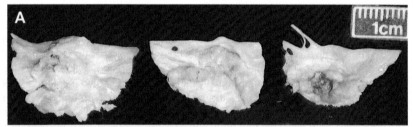
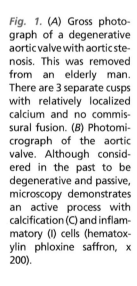
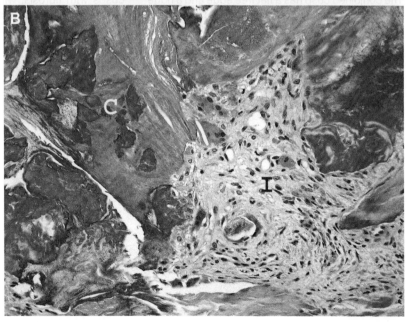

of each cusp. Traditionally, valve calcification was thought to be passive in nature representing dystrophic calcification of degenerated material. The process of valve calcification is an active process with much in common with atherosclerosis and bone formation.[14–16] By histology, calcified valves commonly have calcium, bone, neovascularization, and inflammation (see Fig. 1B).[16,17] Amyloid may also be found in valves, most commonly those with aortic stenosis or mitral stenosis. It may be incidental or form nodules. Valve involvement is recognized in primary AL amyloidosis. Other valve amyloid is not able to be immunotyped.

Degenerative aortic valve stenosis is commonly seen in individuals over age 50 years. Earlier calcification is seen if the valve has been damaged, such as previous surgical manipulation or radiation. Patients with hyperparathyroidism and chronic renal failure patients, especially those who are dialysis dependent, have accelerated valve disease.[18] Some storage diseases, such as certain types of Gaucher's disease, lead to aortic valve disease in young individuals.[19]

CONGENITALLY BICUSPID AORTIC VALVE

Congenitally bicuspid valve is present in 1 to 2% of the population. Some of these valves calcify and are stenotic, while others become regurgitant.[20] The bicuspid valve occurs as two of the cusps fail to split (Fig. 2). The resulting cusp is termed the conjoined cusp. The two congenitally bicuspid valve cusps are usually similar in the circumference they occupy in the aorta, but are rarely equal. The conjoined cusp has a flat free edge and a ridge at the base of the cusp near the aorta. This ridge is perpendicular to the aorta and is termed the raphe. This represents the area of failed cusp division.

The raphe usually extends about half way up the cusp, is of variable size and shape, and often is fibrotic or calcified.

Congenitally bicuspid valve may be associated with an aortopathy, as the ascending aorta and the aortic valve have a similar embryologic origin and development. In a patient with a congenitally bicuspid valve the aorta must be observed for dilatation, as there is a risk of aneurysm or dissection.[21,22] It is not uncommon to receive segments of ascending aorta with a congenitally bicuspid valve specimen.

Congenitally unicuspid valves are usually stenotic and are invariably symptomatic early (Fig. 3). There is failure of the cusps to split and one observes a valve with a tear drop like orifice (unicuspid unicommissural valve), or with no commissures as a dome or hole shaped valve (unicuspid acommissural valve).

POST-INFLAMMATORY–RHEUMATIC AORTIC STENOSIS

Rheumatic valve disease, from chronic complications of rheumatic fever, is the disease most associated with "post-inflammatory" valve disease. The acute rheumatic valve is not seen by the pathologist, but chronically scarred, inflamed valves are seen. Chronically, rheumatic fever leads to neovascularization, chronic inflammation, commissural fusion, valve thickening and calcification. Once the valve is inflamed and there is neovascularization, lymphocytes can infiltrate the valve.[23]

Grossly chronic rheumatic aortic valves have 3 cusps with fibrosis, with or without calcification. The commissures are often fused (Fig. 4). Valves may be thickened and show scar retraction resulting in a combination of aortic stenosis and

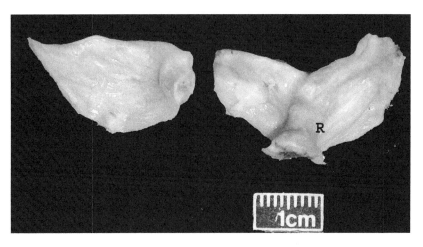

Fig. 2. Gross photograph of a stenotic congenitally bicuspid aortic valve. The cusp size is approximately equal and there is fibrosis and calcium. The cusp on the right has the raphe (R). This is calcified and extends partway up the cusp with its origin at the cusp base. The edge of the cusp is flat and not significantly indented. There is no commissural fusion.

Fig. 3. Gross photograph of a stenotic congenitally unicuspid aortic valve. The valve is significantly calcified and was removed from a young individual with aortic stenosis. This is a unicommissural unicuspid valve.

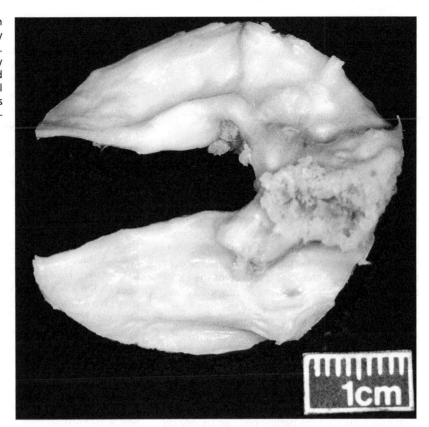

Fig. 4. Rheumatic aortic stenosis: Gross photograph of a stenotic post-inflammatory aortic valve from a patient with a prior history of rheumatic fever. The three cusps are fibrotic and calcified and fused at each commissure producing a valve that is both stenotic and regurgitant, not unusual for a rheumatic valve.

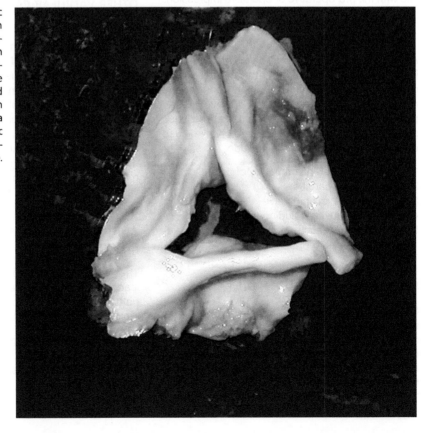

△△ **Differential Diagnosis**
AORTIC VALVE STENOSIS

1. Calcific degeneration-age related degenerative changes

2. Post-inflammatory changes–rheumatic

3. Congenitally bicuspid valve

regurgitation.[12] If the cusps fuse into an acquired bicuspid valve the distinction from a congenitally bicuspid valve is sometimes difficult. In a post-inflammatory fused cusp, one fused cusp should be twice the circumference and size of the other cusp, as it represents fusion of two previously normally sized cusps. The free edge of the fused cusp usually is "v" shaped rather than flat. No raphe is seen. If there is a ridge in the area of commissural fusion, this ridge often extends all the way to the cusp free edge. Sectioning with use of an elastic stain may be useful in the distinction.[8]

Sometimes heavily calcified valves are removed in many pieces due to a difficult surgical excision. In such cases the best the pathologist can usually do is to diagnose calcific valve stenosis and try to correlate with the pre-operative or operative impression.

AORTIC VALVE REGURGITATION OVERVIEW

Aortic valve regurgitation may be due to abnormalities of the aortic valve cusps or the aortic root. The most common mechanisms that cause valve regurgitation are aortic annular dilatation, cusp prolapse, scar retraction of the cusps, and cusp perforation.[21,24] The most common valve cusp causes of aortic regurgitation include:

1. Rheumatic–post-inflammatory changes
2. Infective endocarditis
3. Congenitally bicuspid valve
4. Iatrogenic causes including valvuloplasty
5. Cusp prolapse–such as prolapse into an adjacent ventricular septal defect.

CONGENITALLY BICUSPID VALVE

Some congenitally bicuspid valves become soft and myxoid. These are often associated with aortic dilation and the cusps may have a thickened free edge.[20] A variant type of bicuspid valve, termed the "atypical" variant, has been described to account for up to 3 to 24% of bicuspid valves.[25] This variant has a fenestrated raphe on the conjoined cusp so that there is continuity between the conjoined cusp sinuses. The resulting raphal chord is often only a few mm in thickness. Rarely such a raphe may rupture giving rise to acute aortic regurgitation. Raphal remnants must be distinguished from the residua of cusp perforations secondary to infective endocarditis, and from valve fenestrations. The raphe remnant may also be misinterpreted as a vegetation or thrombus since the clinical situation is acute aortic insufficiency with a valve mass.

POST-INFLAMMATORY–RHEUMATIC VALVES

Post-inflammatory cusp disease produces fibrosis, calcification and commissural fusion of the cusps.[24] However, the fusion and cusp immobility fix the valve orifice open. Rheumatic disease may give a valve that is mixed in regurgitation and stenosis (see **Fig. 4**). Radiation may produce significant cusp fibrosis and retraction of the cusps.[26] Systemic lupus erythematosis (SLE) may scar the cusps with cusp retraction, poor opposition and regurgitation. Aortitis may cause root dilation and regurgitation but some types of aortitis, such as that seen in syphilis and ankylosing spondylitis, may scar or alter the cusps.

OTHER VALVULAR CAUSES OF AORTIC REGURGITATION

Infective endocarditis may cause destruction of the cusps as the infected thrombi, known as vegetations, destroy the cusps leading to defects, erosions, acquired aneurysms that may eventually perforate and leave a hole in the cusp (**Fig. 5**).[9,10] Healed infective endocarditis may leave large defects or valve irregularities.[24] Valvuloplasty of the aortic valve is not common, but when done, the cusps may be torn. A normal aortic valve may prolapse into an adjacent membranous ventricular septal defect (VSD).

AORTIC CAUSES OF AORTIC VALVE REGURGITATION

The other category of conditions commonly leading to aortic valve regurgitation has the pathology in the aortic root, not in the valve cusps.[21,22,24] These aortic diseases include:

- Age-related and hypertension related aortic medial degeneration
- Connective tissue disorders such as Marfan's and Ehlars Danlos
- Aortic dissection
- Aortitis.

Fig. 5. Gross photograph of an aortic valve with regurgitation due to cusp perforation from prior infective endocarditis, after the infection heals, holes and defects may result in a leaky valve.

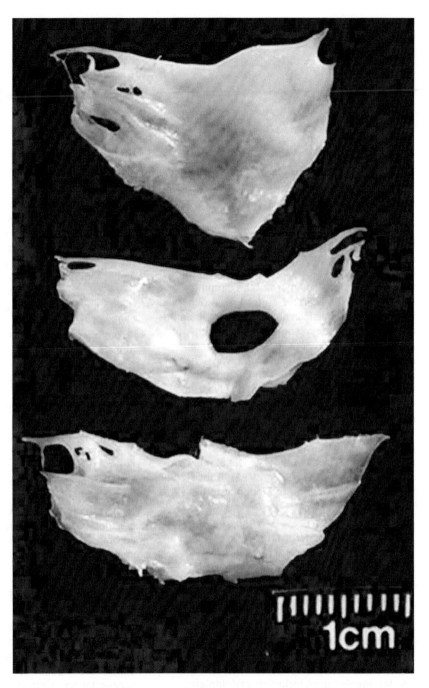

Diseases that produce aortic dilatation include cystic medial necrosis (medial degenerative changes), forms of congenital heart disease, and aortitis. The aorta progressively dilates due to loss of normal collagenous and elastic framework.

Aortic root disorders and dilatation are becoming more common. This probably has to do with improved survival of patients with systemic arterial hypertension, increasing population age, and improving survival of adult congenital heart disease patients.

The valve cusps stretch as the aorta and the aortic root dilate. This is manifest grossly as thin or myxomatous cusps with rolled edges due to chronic hemodynamic insufficiency (**Fig. 6**).[24] In aortitis, the cusps may fibrose and scar. In type A dissection, the aortic valve may be dehisced from the aortic root either by the dissection or the thrombus in the false lumen.

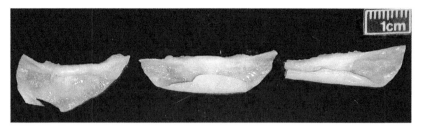

Fig. 6. Gross photograph of a chronically regurgitant aortic valve. The 3 cusps are soft and the chief pathology was in a dilated aorta, rather than intrinsic cusp pathology. Due to chronic regurgitation the free edges of the cusps focally thicken and appear rolled.

MITRAL VALVE ANATOMY

The mitral valve is an atrioventricular valve with leaflets and chordae which attach to papillary muscles and the left ventricle wall. There are two leaflets-the anterior and the posterior. Although the posterior occupies more of the circumference of the annulus, the actual surface area occupied by each of the leaflets is about equal, as the anterior leaflet is longer in length. On either side of the leaflets there are commissures, the posteromedial and the anterolateral. The mitral valve has no septal chordal attachments. The anterior leaflet is in fibrous continuity with the aortic valve.

The leaflets have free edges and closing margins approximately a few mm from the edge. The mitral valve annulus is usually evident. The posterior leaflet has 3 variably formed scallops (P1, P2 and P3) and the anterior leaflet has corresponding regions (A1, A2, and A3). These small indentations allow some redundancy to the valve which is important for competency. The chordae are complex and different surgical classifications exist. The chords are responsible for different functions. Some are important in the basic integrity and structure of the valve, some ensure good leaflet coaptation, while others prevent leaflet prolapse. Rupture of a chord may have very different consequences depending upon the type involved.

The chords attach to two left ventricle papillary muscles, the anterolateral and the posteromedial papillary muscles. The anterior muscle usually has one head while the posteromedial papillary muscle is usually bifid.

Microscopically the valve leaflets have 3 layers: the fibrosa, ventricularis, and the spongiosa.[11] The central fibrosa is responsible for structural support and thus is composed of collagen, and elastic fibers. The fibrosa is covered by the spongiosa on the atrial aspect of the leaflet and the ventricularis on the ventricular aspect. The spongiosa contains proteoglycans, sparse elastic fibers, collagen, and connective tissue cells such as fibroblasts, and valve interstitial cells. On the proximal mitral valve, the spongiosa also contains left atrial cardiac myocytes.

MITRAL STENOSIS OVERVIEW

Mitral stenosis is usually due to leaflet fibrosis, commissural fusion and calcification. Almost all cases are post-inflammatory, usually rheumatic.[27] Other rare causes of mitral stenosis include congenital valve stenosis, storage diseases and medication-related pathology.

RHEUMATIC MITRAL STENOSIS

Rheumatic fever is a late inflammatory non-suppurative complication of pharyngitis caused by Group A beta-hemolytic Streptococci. The pathogenesis of rheumatic fever relates to humoral and cellular mediated immune responses with development of autoimmunity.[28] Products of the Streptococcus have "molecular mimicry" to

---

△△ ***Differential Diagnosis***
AORTIC VALVE
REGURGITATION

Valve cusp pathology

1. Rheumatic–post-inflammatory changes

2. Post-infective endocarditis

3. Congenitally bicuspid valve

4. Iatrogenic causes including vavluloplasty

5. Cusp prolapse – VSD related

Aortic root pathology

1. Age-related medial degeneration

2. Marfan's and other connective tissue diseases

3. Aortic dissection

4. Aortitis

human tissue and are recognized by the immune system, thus initiating an autoimmune response. Individuals develop antibodies to the carbohydrate and the M protein of the Streptococcal organism. The anti-carbohydrate antibodies cross react with the valvular endothelium producing injury and allow entry of inflammatory cells responsible for local cytokine release, and interstitial cell damage with neovascularization and chronic inflammation.[1] The M-protein antibodies have molecular mimicry with myosin. Cardiac myosin is not present in the valve, but laminin links myosin in the valve. The anti-myosin antibody recognizes laminin, part of the valve basement membrane structure.[28,29]

The acute involvement of the heart in rheumatic fever is pancarditis with inflammation of the myocardium, pericardium and endocardium. In acute disease, thrombi form along the lines of valve closure. These small thrombi have been termed "verrucous" endocarditis and do not produce valve destruction. The leaflets may have associated edema and inflammatory cell infiltration.[23,30] Such acute diseased valves are not surgical specimens.

The valves most affected by rheumatic fever are the mitral, aortic, tricuspid and pulmonary, in that order. The chronically scarred, inflamed and neo-vascularized valve is commonly encountered by the surgical pathologist.[1,31] The mechanism of stenosis is due to leaflet fibrosis, calcification, commissural fusion, chordal fusion and shortening (Fig. 7). Valve leaflets may be thickened and show scar retraction. The chordae are often thick and shortened. The subvalvular chordal space may seem to disappear with short thick chords attached almost directly to the papillary muscles (see Fig. 7C). The subvalvular apparatus pathology can be graded by echocardiography and the results used to plan valve surgery or interventional procedures.[32,33] At the commissures of mitral valves there is often loss of surface endothelium with erosion and overlying thrombus material. Histology shows neo-vascularization, chronic inflammation and fibrosis with alteration and damage of the underlying valve architecture. Large fibrous endocardial onlays are present on microscopic examination.

Rare causes of mitral valve stenosis include storage diseases and medication-related pathology, especially ergot and migraine medications. Ergotamine associated valve disease chiefly affects the mitral valve and produces pathology similar to carcinoid valve disease. Valve leaflets are typically very thick with chordal fusion and shortening and commissural fusion. Large myofibroblast rich plaques are stuck on the underlying valve proper without underlying valve leaflet destruction.[34,35]

The secondary effects of mitral valve stenosis upon the heart involve the left atrium and the right heart. Chronically as the left atrium enlarges, the myocytes undergo degenerative changes and the atrium is prone to fibrillation. Atrial fibrillation surgery may include excision of atrium segments, incision or radiofrequency ablation. Pieces of atrium including the appendage or thrombus often accompany surgically excised rheumatic mitral valves.

MITRAL INSUFFICIENCY OVERVIEW

The mitral valve apparatus is a complicated structure and the leaflets, annulus, chordae, papillary muscles and even the left ventricle all must work together to ensure valve normal function. Different diseases affect multiple parts of the valve. An organized method of categorizing causes of mitral insufficiency is to consider each anatomic structure separately.

LEAFLET CAUSES OF MITRAL REGURGITATION

Abnormalities of the leaflet causing regurgitation include[9]:

- Perforation (post infective endocarditis)
- Scar retraction (post-inflammatory-often rheumatic)
- Medications (anorectic drugs)
- The degenerative floppy mitral valve (myxomatous degeneration).

Myxomatous Valve Disease

Myxomatous valve degeneration may be a degenerative age related change or seen in association with syndromes such as Marfan's, Ehlers Danlos or osteogenesis imperfecta. Surgical pathology examination does not allow discrimination between these different pathoetiologies. Most myxomatous degeneration is age related in nature. Myxomatous valves are large redundant, thickened, "floppy" valves with endocardial fibrous thickening and accumulation of ground substances (glycosaminoglycans) in the valve spongiosa layer (Fig. 8).[36–38] The myxomatous change is most common in the posterior leaflet and the process may be very marked in just one scallop. Anterior leaflet degeneration occurs less commonly. The entire valve may be severely involved with large thick redundant leaflets (termed Barlow's disease). Commissures are not fused. Chordae may be ruptured. Calcification is not common in the leaflet but it may be seen in accompanying annular tissues.[31]

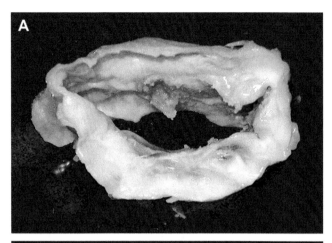

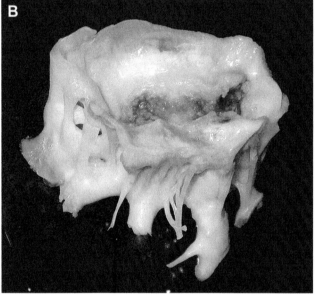

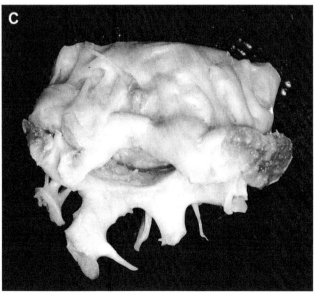

Fig. 7. (A) Gross photograph of a stenotic post-inflammatory mitral valve in an individual with a history of rheumatic fever. The leaflets are fibrotic and calcified and the commissures fused rendering the valve stenotic. It is not unusual for the calcium to ulcerate and thrombus may attach. (B) Gross photograph of a stenotic rheumatic mitral valve. The chordae are significantly fibrotic and thickened. Leaflet calcium and fibrosis are also evident. (C) Gross photograph of a chronic rheumatic mitral valve with stenosis. The photograph from the underside of the valve demonstrates the marked sub-leaflet fibrosis and fused chordae. The fusion has lessened the distance between the papillary muscles and the leaflets.

Fig. 8. (*A*) Gross photograph of an excised portion of a myxomatous mitral valve "floppy" mitral valve. The valve is thickened but soft. As is usually the case, only part of the valve has actually been excised. (*B*) Photomicrograph of a myxomatous mitral valve demonstrating the bluish colored deposits of matrix material in the valve spongiosa layer (Movat pentachrome, x 200).

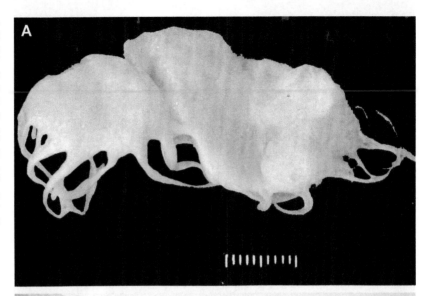

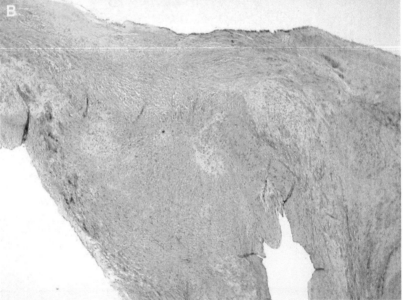

Mitral valve repair is the procedure of choice in the surgical treatment of degenerative mitral regurgitation. Mitral valve repair usually consists of correcting the specific component of the mitral apparatus responsible for the abnormal coaptation leading to regurgitation, and remodeling and stabilizing the mitral annulus by the placement of an annular ring or band. Asymmetric leaflet prolapse from redundant leaflet tissue or ruptured chords can be managed by resection of portion of the posterior mitral leaflet. If the anterior mitral leaflet is involved, chordal reconstruction using chordal transfer or artificial chords can be performed. Some form of annuloplasty is then performed to remodel the annulus and to support the leaflet repair.[39] With repair the surgical pathologist usually receives small pieces of leaflets and chordae, rather than an entire valve (see **Fig. 8**C, D).[31] Despite the specimen small size, microscopy usually demonstrates the myxomatous changes.

Infective Endocarditis

Infective endocarditis may lead to leaflet and chordal destruction (**Fig. 9**).[9,10] The infection may weaken the leaflet tissue leading to pouches or aneurysms (**Fig. 10**). In the process of healing, or if the infection continues, the aneurysm may become like a sieve due to perforation. Infected thrombi may also destroy the chords and cause

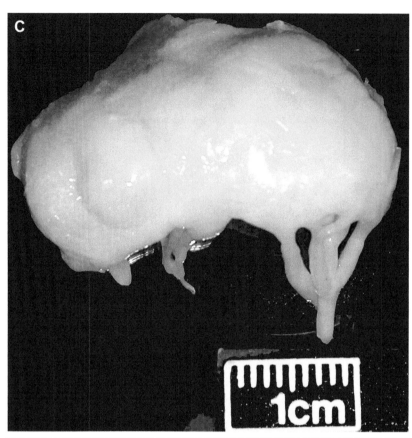

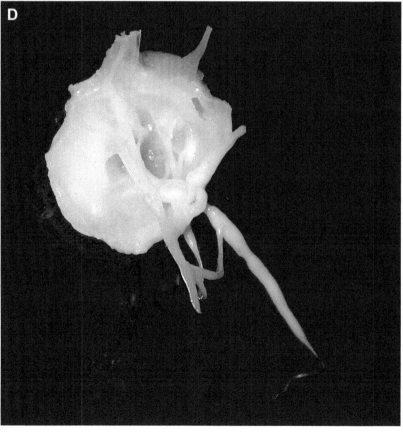

Fig. 8. (*C*) Gross photograph of an excised portion of a myxomatous mitral valve- "floppy" mitral valve. This is a very typical specimen derived from excision of a scallop of the posterior leaflet during valve repair. (*D*) Gross photograph of an excised portion of a myxomatous mitral valve- "floppy" mitral valve. Another portion of posterior leaflet with chordal thinning and chordal entanglement close to the leaflet. These changes are highly suggestive of prior chordal rupture.

Fig. 9. Excised anterior mitral leaflet with vegetations on the leaflet and chordae from infective endocarditis. Tissue destruction has necessitated valve replacement.

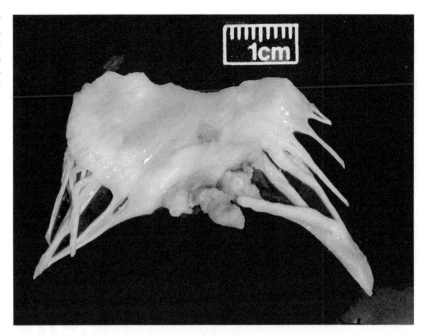

them to rupture. Chronically the infections may lead to leaflet and chordal loss with valve defects and holes. Fibrotic changes may thicken the leaflets and they may be retracted leading to incomplete coaptation. Valve repair may be attempted acutely or chronically (**Fig. 11**).

Drug Related Valve Pathology

Medications, including anorexogenic drugs (fenfluramine-phentermine), ergotamine and methy-sergide (migraine medications) have been described as producing carcinoid like valve disease. The mechanism of valve injury is thought to be activation of the 5HT-2B receptors. The combination of fenfluramine and phentermine (Fen-Phen) was introduced in North America in the mid 1990s. Connolly and colleagues[40] reported heart valve disease shortly thereafter in 1997. There is still some debate as to the actual risk and incidence of the valvulopathy associated with anorexogenic agents, but it is probably low.[41]

Fig. 10. Excised mitral valve tissue with chronic leaflet perforation and detached perforated aneurysm. These lesions related to infective endocarditis render the valve regurgitant.

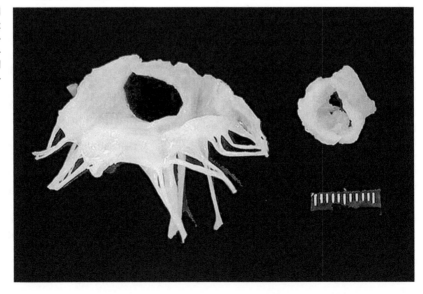

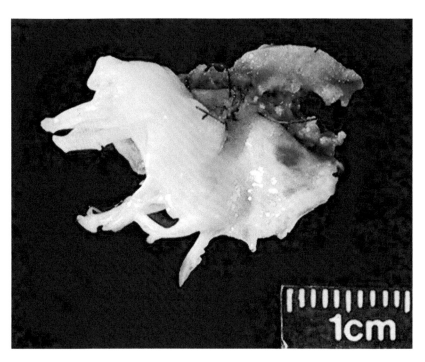

Fig. 11. Excised portion of mitral valve with damage from infective endocarditis. There has been attempted repair of the defect, as noted by the sutures. If the surgeon is not satisfied with the repair, the pathologist may receive the valve with repair sequelae.

Grossly and microscopically the valve disease or valvulopathy associated with anorexogenic drugs has been reported to be similar morphologically to that of carcinoid valve disease.[40,42] The left sided valves are predominantly affected. White plaques are noted grossly and there may be chordal encasement and fusion, but not rupture. The commissures are not fused, in contrast to rheumatic disease. Doming or hooding of the mitral leaflets is not seen, in contrast to floppy valve disease. By microscopic examination, the valves have myofibroblast and glycosaminoglycan rich endocardial lesions with preservation of the underlying valve architecture. These lesions are onlays of glycosaminoglycan, collagen, and myofibroblasts that are superficial to the valve elastic membrane, but deep to the surface endothelium. The valve proper may have myxoid degeneration with accumulation of glycosaminoglycans. The onlays also may contain chronic inflammatory cells and there is neovascularization within the onlay lesions and in the valve proper.[43] Similar carcinoid-like valve disease has also been noted recently with Pergolide, an ergot derived dopamine receptor agonist used for treatment of Parkinson's disease.[44,45]

CHORDAL CAUSES OF MITRAL REGURGITATION

Chordal abnormities causing regurgitation are due to chordal elongation, as observed in a myxomatous floppy valve, or actual chordal rupture from a floppy valve or after infective endocarditis. In elongation and myxomatous change, the regurgitation is chronic. In rupture the regurgitation is sudden leading to acute ventricle dilatation and marked severe left heart failure. Urgent surgical repair may be required.

In myxomatous valves studies have shown structural anomalies in not only the leaflets, but also the chordae.[46,47] These are of abnormal composition and are weak and prone to elongation and rupture. One should examine the chordal ends for pointed configurations suggestive of rupture (see **Fig.** 8D). Twisting and entanglement of the chords may occur if the rupture is chronic.[31] By microscopy fibrin may be seen and the area should always be examined for the possibility of infection.

VENTRICULAR CAUSES OF MITRAL REGURGITATION

Left ventricle dilation of any cause (including chronic ischemia or cardiomyopathy) may lead to poor opposition of the mitral leaflets. Abnormal dilatation or fibrosis and calcification of the annulus may lead to mitral regurgitation. Left ventricle dilation may lead to annular dilatation and misalignment of the papillary muscles with leaflet "restriction" due to the geometric distortion of the ventricle. Part of mitral valve repair is to re-establish good contact between the leaflets.

Excised pieces of valve leaflet tissue may show mild degenerative changes (fibrosis, myxomatous change and calcium) and one is often underwhelmed by the pathology until one realizes that the prime pathology is in the ventricle, not in the surgical specimen.

MITRAL ANNULAR CALCIFICATION

Mitral annular calcification (MAC) is a common finding in the hearts of elderly patients. MAC is probably a pathologic process due to degenerative changes in the mitral annulus. Although it is considered as a cause for mitral regurgitation, when moderate or greater mitral regurgitation is present in a patient with MAC, it is important to look for another cause before ascribing the mitral regurgitation to the presence of MAC. MAC can co-exist with sclerotic changes of the mitral leaflets, which are thickened and retracted.[48] MAC is often associated with myxomatous degeneration of the mitral valve leaflets and in fact some think the leaflet disorder puts stress on the annulus causing it to secondarily degenerate. The annular calcium is localized to the posterior mitral ring but the calcium may extend onto the leaflet, fixing it and producing leaflet immobility. It also may liquefy and form a left atrial posterior wall mass that can be confused with a granuloma or an abscess. MAC may also ulcerate with thrombus deposition.[49]

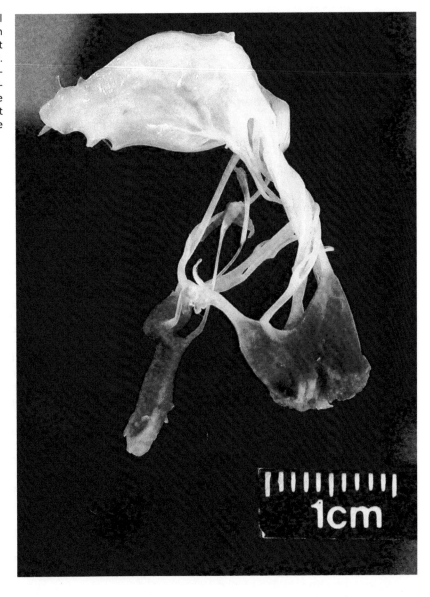

Fig. 12. Excised mitral valve tissue with an attached infarcted left ventricle papillary muscle. This excision was necessary for acute mitral regurgitation due to muscle rupture. The valve leaflet is usually unremarkable in such cases.

PAPILLARY MUSCLE CAUSES OF MITRAL REGURGITATION

The left ventricle papillary muscles may become dysfunctional from ischemia or infarction. With acute ischemia the muscles may temporarily stop contracting, a process known as stunning. With heart failure and chronic ischemia the myocytes may undergo degenerative myocytolysis and lose their myofilaments reverting to a more primitive phenotype for survival. This is known as hibernating myocardium and it also is non-contractile.

In acute myocardial infarction the muscles may infarct and die. This dead muscle is no longer contractile. In the most dramatic manifestation, the papillary muscle may rupture leading to acute mitral regurgitation (Fig. 12). Mitral valve replace-ment is often necessary and the excised leaflet tissue may be normal.

When a myocardial infarct heals, the papillary muscle may fibrose and become non-contractile. Scar retraction and underlying ventricular distortion and dilatation from the infarct may distort or restrict the normal mitral valve architecture. Displacement of the papillary muscles in the setting of left ventricular dilatation can also cause improper mitral leaflet coaptation and mitral regurgitation (as discussed in ventricular cases of mitral regurgitation).

Surgical pathologists usually only receive papillary muscles after they are acutely ruptured after infarction. In chronic "ischemic regurgitation" the excised valve leaflets may be normal or only show age related changes. Correlation with the clinical history helps clear the confusion.

Differential Diagnosis
MITRAL VALVE INSUFFICIENCY AS GROUPED BY ANATOMIC SITE

Leaflets

1. Perforation–post infective endocarditis

2. Scar retraction–post-inflammatory causes–rheumatic

3. Medications–Phen Fen

4. Floppy mitral valve – myxomatous degeneration

Chordae

1. Elongation–floppy valve

2. Rupture–floppy valve or post-infective endocarditis

Mitral annulus

1. Left ventricular dilatation related

2. Mitral annular calcification

Left ventricle - dilatation

1. Ischemia

2. Cardiomyopathy

Papillary muscles

1. Ischemia-related dysfunction–acute or chronic

2. Infarct–necrosis or fibrosis

3. Post-infarct rupture

TRICUSPID AND PULMONARY VALVES OVERVIEW

The tricuspid and pulmonic valves are not common surgical specimens, as compared with the mitral and aortic valves. The tricuspid and pulmonary valves may become both stenotic or regurgitant. Congenital anomalies, infective endocarditis and carcinoid disease account for most surgically excised specimens.

TRICUSPID VALVE ANATOMY

The tricuspid valve is an atrioventricular valve with three leaflets:

1. Anterior
2. Septal
3. Posterior.

The anterior leaflet is the largest of the three. As with all cardiac valves, there is a free edge and a line of closure, located on the atrial side of the tricuspid valve. There are three commissures separating the leaflets. Each leaflet has chordae attaching to ventricular papillary muscles and there are septal leaflet chordae that attach directly to the underlying adjacent ventricular septum.

The anterior papillary muscle is large and has multiple heads, as is also common with the posterior muscle. The annulus of the tricuspid valve is discontinuous and not as well formed as the mitral annulus. The tricuspid valve is separate from the pulmonary valve due to the presence of the infundibular septum of the morphologic right ventricle.

PULMONARY VALVE ANATOMY

The pulmonary valve is a semilunar valve. The valve has a corona shaped annulus. There are 3 cusps separated from each other at 3 commissures. The cusps are the anterior, and behind the anterior are the left and right cusps. The cusps have a free edge and a line of closure along the ventricular surface. The cusps are thinner than the aortic valve cusps.

TRICUSPID VALVE REGURGITATION

Tricuspid regurgitation is very common, often functional from left heart failure leading to pulmonary hypertension and right ventricular dysfunction and dilatation. In this setting, the tricuspid valve is morphologically normal but the tricuspid annulus is enlarged causing incomplete leaflet coaptation.

Rheumatic involvement of tricuspid valve is rare but can occur usually with co-existent mitral valve disease.[50,51] The changes of the tricuspid leaflet resemble those of the mitral leaflet, namely the leaflet and/or chords are thickened with restriction in excursion and incomplete coaptation of the leaflets.

Flail of the tricuspid leaflet is caused by a ruptured chord or a ruptured papillary muscle. Closed chest trauma can lead to papillary muscle rupture and flail of the tricuspid leaflet.[52–55] Another cause is right ventricular myocardial biopsy which inadvertently damages the papillary muscle or chord resulting in flail of the tricuspid leaflet.[56,57] Other causes of tricuspid regurgitation are infective endocarditis and Ebstein's anomaly.[58–60]

EBSTEIN'S ANOMALY

Ebstein's anomaly is an important valvular cause of tricuspid regurgitation. Normally the atrioventricular valves delaminate from their underlying developing ventricle. Failure to delaminate causes the valve leaflets to become elongated and only come off the wall of the ventricle close to the apex. The right atrium seems huge (in reality it usually is) and the ventricle has "atrialized." The valve leaflets are not well formed and are dysplastic (**Fig. 13**).[61] The posterior and septal leaflets are chiefly affected by the apical displacement and the anterior leaflet often is the most dysplastic. The anterior leaflet may be large, thick, abnormally formed and with multiple orifices and defects. The chordae are often short and thick. Underneath the leaflets the right ventricle undergoes eccentric hypertrophy from volume overload and chronic regurgitation.

CARCINOID VALVE DISEASE

Carcinoid valve disease most commonly affects the tricuspid and the pulmonary valves.[62] The disease is commonly related to metastatic carcinoid tumor in the liver usually from a metastatic primary in the gastrointestinal tract. Carcinoid valve disease is postulated to relate to increased serum levels of serotonin which induces TGF (transforming growth factor) beta expression in the valve via serotonin 5HT-2A and 5HT-2B receptors.[63,64] TGF beta induces valvular endothelial

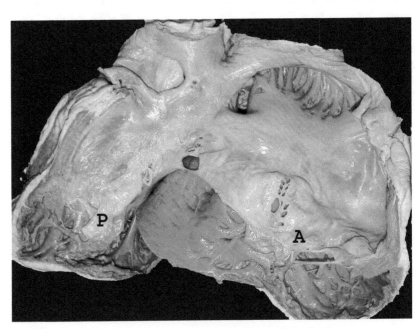

Fig. 13. This heart has been opened to demonstrate the typical pathology seen in Ebstein's anomaly. The leaflets are relatively fixed to the underlying endocardium. The anterior leaflet is thickened, redundant and has accessory orifices. Such valves are regurgitant. They are occasionally excised but there are also efforts made for valve repair. A, anterior leaflet; P, posterior leaflet.

cells and interstitial cells to trans-differentiate into myofibroblasts which produce the characteristic carcinoid valve plaques.[65,66]

The affected valves are white and thickened grossly (Fig. 14A). The thickening is due to fibromuscular plaques or onlays. The plaques involve the cusps of the semilunar valves and the leaflets, chords and papillary muscles of the atrioventricular valves. The endocardial plaques cause valve thickening and retraction leading to valvular regurgitation and stenosis. Regurgitant valves are most common, with mixed pulmonary stenosis and pulmonary insufficiency and tricuspid insufficiency.

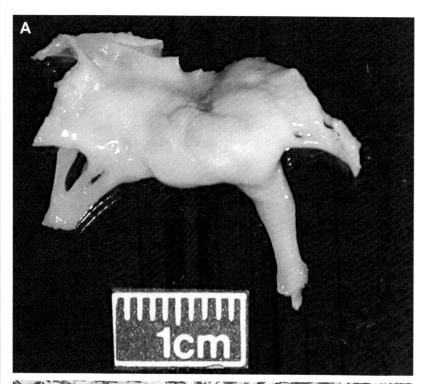

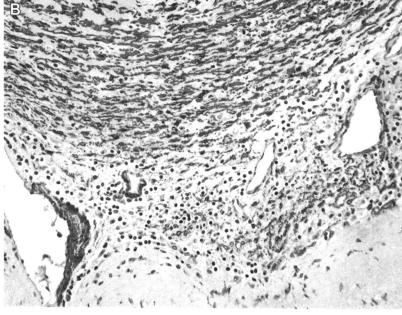

Fig. 14. (*A*) Excised portion of tricuspid valve leaflet from an individual with carcinoid valve disease. The leaflet and chordae are both thickened and white appearing. (*B*) Photomicrograph of carcinoid plaque demonstrating brown staining of the myofibroblasts and smooth muscle of the onlays (immunostain muscle specific actin x 200).

The valve thickening is due to proliferation of myofibroblast like cells and accumulation of extracellular matrix in the endocardial onlay plaque valvular lesions. Carcinoid plaques do not destroy the underlying valve architecture. Immunostains for smooth muscle actin or muscle specific actin outline the plaques well (see **Fig. 14B**).

TRICUSPID VALVE STENOSIS

Tricuspid stenosis may be congenital and may be associated with a dysplastic valve.[67] Acquired stenosis is usually rheumatic and is invariably associated with concomitant left sided valve disease. Fungal endocarditis with large vegetations may cause valve stenosis due to the large size of the vegetations. Indwelling catheters, shunt lines, pacemakers and defibrillators leads may incorporate into the valve leaflets or chords, but unless associated with thrombus they do not usually cause significant valve destruction or stenosis. Some lines are associated with calcific masses termed calcified amorphous tumors.[68] These pseudotumors probably represent calcified thrombus and are also associated with coagulation disorders such as lupus anticoagulant.

UNICUSPID AND BICUSPID PULMONARY VALVES

Unicuspid and bicuspid pulmonary valves may be isolated or associated with syndromes including Tetralogy of Fallot and Noonan's syndrome.[69]

Unicuspid valves are acommissural dome shaped or unicommissural teardrop shaped, analogous to their aortic counterparts. Raphes may be present in both variants. These valves are stenotic and usually symptomatic after a time. Traditionally they were replaced, but now are repaired with valvuloplasty or stented (including percutaneous stenting) with reasonable results. Bicuspid pulmonary valves may be asymptomatic and may be regurgitant or stenotic. These are more common than unicuspid valves. There are also quadricuspid pulmonary valves which are usually competent or at least minimally symptomatic. These unicuspid and bicuspid pulmonary valves are only usually surgical specimens if excised during surgery for congenital heart disease (**Fig. 15**).

TRICUSPID AND PULMONIC VALVE INFECTIVE ENDOCARDITIS

Right sided tricuspid or pulmonary valve infective endocarditis may be associated with indwelling lines or catheters, pacemakers or defibrillator lead infections, intravenous drug use, or TPN.[70] The valve destruction is more clinically silent than left sided valve disease, with the development of progressive right heart failure and pulmonary manifestations including pulmonary emboli and infarcts, pulmonary abscesses, empyema, pleuritis and effusions.

Bacterial and fungal infections are both common in these valves, probably reflecting the origin of the infections or the underlying condition

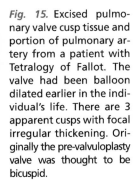

Fig. 15. Excised pulmonary valve cusp tissue and portion of pulmonary artery from a patient with Tetralogy of Fallot. The valve had been balloon dilated earlier in the individual's life. There are 3 apparent cusps with focal irregular thickening. Originally the pre-valvuloplasty valve was thought to be bicuspid.

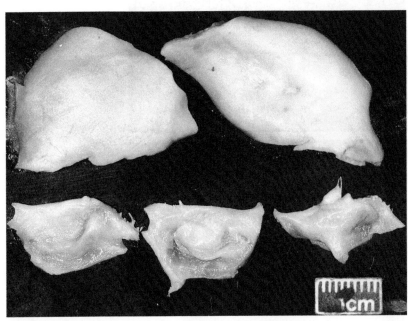

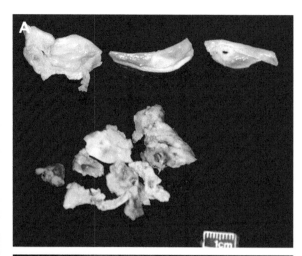

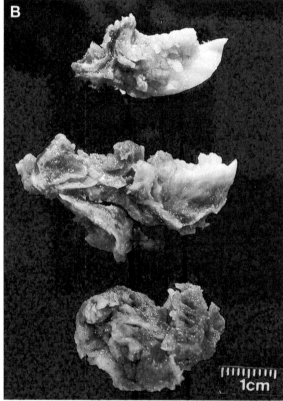

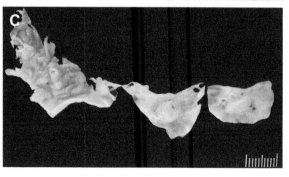

Fig. 16. (A) Excised pulmonary valve and some tricuspid valve tissue from a patient with right sided infective endocarditis. The pulmonary valve on top has cusp destruction and a cusp perforation. The lower tricuspid valve tissue is not recognizable as it is mostly obscured by infected vegetation material. (B) Excised aortic valve with severe infective endocarditis and cusp destruction by infected vegetations. (C) Excised aortic valve with chronic damage from prior endocarditis. There is cusp destruction of the left cusp and formation of an aneurysm in the center cusp. Some of these aneurysms rupture and become perforations.

or situation associated with the endocarditis.[71,72] Vegetations in right sided endocarditis may be large and obstructive (**Fig. 16A**).

INFECTIVE ENDOCARDITIS OVERVIEW

Infective endocarditis (IE) may give rise to numerous extracardiac, cardiac and valvular findings including infected thrombi (vegetations), sequelae of local tissue destruction, and systemic manifestations including vasculitis, emboli and ischemic events. Endocarditis is best described by its anatomic location and the organism involved. Infective endocarditis may arise in normal hearts with normal valves, or more commonly in patients with abnormal cardiac anatomy.[10,73]

ACTIVE INFECTIVE ENDOCARDITIS VALVE PATHOLOGY

On gross examination, infected thrombi of variable size, commonly known as "vegetations," are detected along the lines of valve closure or at the low pressure end of jet lesions.[10,74] They are usually gray, pink, or brown and are often friable. IE vegetations may be located anywhere on the valve cusp or leaflet or endocardial surface. In fact, this is an important feature, as valve thrombi associated with non-bacterial thrombotic endocarditis (NBTE) and those related to rheumatic fever do not have

Key Features
VALVE PATHOLOGY OF
INFECTIVE ENDOCARDITIS

Acute endocarditis

- Vegetations-infected thrombi
- Valve ulcers or erosions
- Aneurysms
- Chord ruptures
- Annular and ring abscess
- Endocardial jet lesions
- Flail leaflet or cusps

Chronic or healed endocarditis

- Perforations
- Calcified nodules
- Valve cusp or leaflet defects
- Valve fibrosis and scarring

this variability in location. Thrombi from NBTE, rheumatic fever, Libman Sacks are not associated with valve destruction. IE vegetations are destructive (see **Fig. 16A, B**).

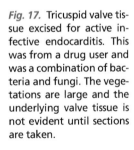
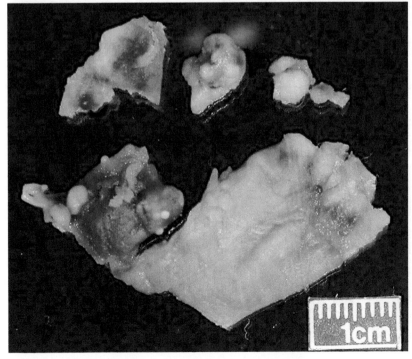

Fig. 17. Tricuspid valve tissue excised for active infective endocarditis. This was from a drug user and was a combination of bacteria and fungi. The vegetations are large and the underlying valve tissue is not evident until sections are taken.

The infected valves may have destructive lesions leading to perforations, defects, aneurysms, erosions and chordal ruptures. Thrombi may obstruct the valvular orifice creating stenosis, although this is rare as most IE causes insufficiency. Chordae may be ruptured resulting in flail leaflets.[75] Leaflet or cusp aneurysms bulge toward the flow surface and may resemble "windsocks." If

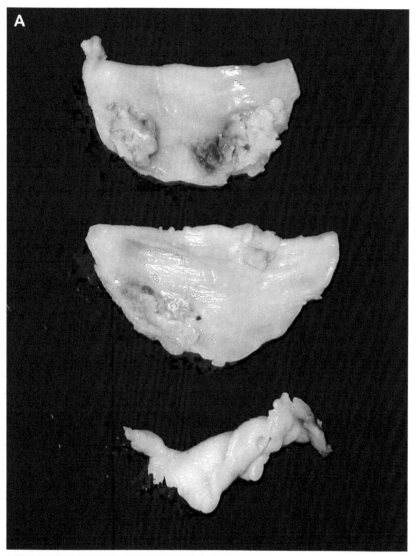

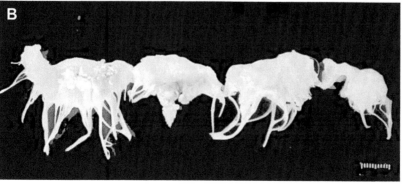

Fig. 18. (A) Healing infective endocarditis of a pulmonary valve. The cusp vegetations are beginning to organize and form nodules. (B) Excised mitral valve with damage from prior infective endocarditis. Chordal destruction and small calcified vegetations are noted.

the aneurysm tip ruptures, the valve may become severely regurgitant due to cusp or leaflet defects (see **Figs. 10** and **16C**).

Early in the disease course, or with very virulent organisms, there are fibrin, neutrophils and clumps of organisms. With therapy, the organisms may calcify and the thrombi organize. Organizing thrombus may show no easily recognizable organisms, and only show acute and chronic inflammation with neovascularization and fibroblastic proliferation. Gram stain may be negative but silver stain may still show organisms.

Fungal endocarditis is usually encountered with intravenous drug use, post surgically, with immunosuppression or in the immunocompromised individual.[76] Intravenous hyper- alimentation, antibiotic therapy, long term venous catheters, pacemakers, defibrillators and other intravascular devices also may contribute to the incidence of fungal IE.[72] The organisms are usually Candida or Aspergillus. Classical clinical manifestations of bacterial IE are often absent. Fungal infected thrombi are usually quite large and friable.[10,77] Valve orifice obstruction and clinical valve stenosis may occur if the size of the thrombus is large (**Fig. 17**).[72,78–80] Diagnosis after an embolic event is not unusual and blood cultures are often negative.[79]

CHRONIC INFECTIVE ENDOCARDITIS PATHOLOGY

With successful medical treatment the infected vegetations may organize and the thrombi may form calcific valve nodules (**Fig. 18**). The valve may have defects at the edges or central defects forming irregular perforations. Around the holes or perforation there may be brown nodules of organisms that eventually form fibrocalcific nodules. Gram stain may be negative but silver stain may still show organisms. The destruction of the valve tissue may lead to defects at the margins with resulting poor valve closure. Chordae may be ruptured resulting in flail leaflets and valve regurgitation. The ruptured chords may knot and calcify along with the organizing infected thrombi. The valve itself may thicken and the chords may fuse. All these are significant contributors to chronic valve regurgitation.

Ventricular papillary muscles may rupture for multiple reasons in IE. The infection may extend from an adjacent chord and cause myocardial necrosis and rupture. A coronary arterial embolus may cause a myocardial infarct with papillary muscle rupture, similar to any acute myocardial infarct. Finally, an embolus may lead to a myocardial abscess with local tissue destruction.

CONCLUSIONS ON EVALUATION OF NATIVE CARDIAC VALVES

Native cardiac valve disease is due to many causes. Careful gross examination remains most valuable for determining the correct diagnosis. Sectioning valves may be contributory in ruling out infection and investigation of unusual valve diseases including storage and drug related disorders. Stenotic valve lesions are usually degenerative or post-inflammatory and not difficult to diagnose. Surgical specimens from regurgitant valve lesions are more complicated as the pathology may be in the valve or in adjacent structures. Excised valve tissue may be unremarkable. Regurgitant lesions may require clinical pathologic correlation for correct diagnosis. It is always important to remain vigilant for the possibly of valve infection.

Mortality and morbidity from valve surgery have continued to improve. The prognosis is often predictable reflecting patient characteristics and risk scoring systems have been developed. There is a trend to repair valves, rather than replace them. This means the surgical pathologist receives less tissue (with more expectations). Future advances will include improvements in valve repair techniques, use of interventional devices for repair, trans-catheter valve procedures and eventually tissue engineered valves.

Pitfalls
SURGICAL VALVE PATHOLOGY ASSESSMENT

! Contamination of a specimen before adequate assessment for the possibility of infection

! Use of swabs rather than submitting infected tissue for culture

! Inadequate gross assessment of the valve specimen

! Failure to assess both sides of the valve surgical specimen

! Poor documentation of gross findings

! Failure to recognize and assess other cardiac tissues submitted with the valve tissue

! Not remembering that the excised valve tissue may be nearly normal in valve repair procedures

! Making a diagnosis of calcification and fibrosis on all valves rather than a pathoetiological diagnosis

REFERENCES

1. Veinot JP. Pathology of inflammatory native valvular heart disease. Cardiovasc Pathol 2006;15:243–51.
2. Stone JR, Basso C, Baandrup UT, et al. Recommendations for processing cardiovascular surgical pathology specimens: a consensus statement from the Standards and Definitions Committee of the Society for Cardiovascular Pathology and the Association for European Cardiovascular Pathology. Cardiovasc Pathol 2012;21:2–16.
3. Bayer AS, Bolger AF, Taubert KA, et al. Diagnosis and management of infective endocarditis and its complications. Circulation 1998;98:2936–48.
4. Baddour LM, Wilson WR, Bayer AS, et al. Infective endocarditis: diagnosis, antimicrobial therapy, and management of complications: a statement for healthcare professionals from the committee on rheumatic Fever, endocarditis, and kawasaki disease, council on cardiovascular disease in the young, and the councils on clinical cardiology, stroke, and cardiovascular surgery and anesthesia, american heart association–executive summary: endorsed by the infectious diseases society of america. Circulation 2005;111:3167–84.
5. Breitkopf C, Hammel D, Scheld HH, et al. Impact of a molecular approach to improve the microbiological diagnosis of infective heart valve endocarditis. Circulation 2005;111:1415–21.
6. Greub G, Lepidi H, Rovery C, et al. Diagnosis of infectious endocarditis in patients undergoing valve surgery. Am J Med 2005;118:230–8.
7. Rice PA, Madico GE. Polymerase chain reaction to diagnose infective endocarditis: will it replace blood cultures? Circulation 2005;111:1352–4.
8. Waller BF, Carter JB, Williams HJ Jr, et al. Bicuspid aortic valve. Comparison of congenital and acquired types. Circulation 1973;48:1140–50.
9. Veinot JP, Walley VM. Focal and patchy cardiac valve lesions: a clinicopathological review. Can J Cardiol 2000;16:1489–507.
10. LeSaux N, Veinot JP, Masters RG, et al. The surgical pathlogy of infective endocarditis. J Surg Path 1997;2:223–32.
11. Dare AJ, Veinot JP, Edwards WD, et al. New observations on the etiology of aortic valve disease: a surgical pathologic study of 236 cases from 1990. Hum Pathol 1993;24:1330–8.
12. Schoen FJ. Cardiac valves and valvular pathology Update on function, disease, repair, and replacement. Cardiovasc Pathol 2005;14:189–94.
13. Subramanian R, Olson LJ, Edwards WD. Surgical pathology of pure aortic stenosis: a study of 374 cases. Mayo Clin Proc 1984;59:683–90.
14. Rajamannan NM, Subramaniam M, Rickard D, et al. Human aortic valve calcification is associated with an osteoblast phenotype. Circulation 2003;107:2181–4.
15. Wallby L, Janerot-Sjoberg B, Steffensen T, et al. T lymphocyte infiltration in non-rheumatic aortic stenosis: a comparative descriptive study between tricuspid and bicuspid aortic valves. Heart 2002;88:348–51.
16. Mohler ER III, Gannon F, Reynolds C, et al. Bone formation and inflammation in cardiac valves. Circulation 2001;103:1522–8.
17. Srivatsa SS, Harrity PJ, Maercklein PB, et al. Increased cellular expression of matrix proteins that regulate mineralization is associated with calcification of native human and porcine xenograft bioprosthetic heart valves. J Clin Invest 1997;99:996–1009.
18. Kajbaf S, Veinot JP, Ha A, et al. Comparison of surgically removed cardiac valves of patients with ESRD with those of the general population. Am J Kidney Dis 2005;46:86–93.
19. Veinot JP, Elstein D, Hanania D, et al. Gaucher's disease with valve calcification: possible role of Gaucher cells, bone matrix proteins and integrins. Can J Cardiol 1999;15:211–6.
20. Sabet HY, Edwards WD, Tazelaar HD, et al. Congenitally bicuspid aortic valves: a surgical pathology study of 542 cases (1991 through 1996) and a literature review of 2,715 additional cases. Mayo Clin Proc 1999;74:14–26.
21. Edwards JE. Lesions causing or simulating aortic insufficiency. Cardiovasc Clin 1973;5:127–48.
22. de Sa M, Moshkovitz Y, Butany J, et al. Histologic abnormalities of the ascending aorta and pulmonary trunk in patients with bicuspid aortic valve disease: clinical relevance to the ross procedure. J Thorac Cardiovasc Surg 1999;118:588–94.
23. Roberto S, Kosanke S, Dunn ST, et al. Pathogenic mechanisms in rheumatic carditis: focus on valvular endothelium. J Infect Dis 2001;183:507–11.
24. Olson LJ, Subramanian R, Edwards WD. Surgical pathology of pure aortic insufficiency: a study of 225 cases. Mayo Clin Proc 1984;59:835–41.
25. Walley VM, Antecol DH, Kyrollos AG, et al. Congenitally bicuspid aortic valves: study of a variant wih fenestrated raphe. Can J Cardiol 1994;10:535–42.
26. Veinot JP, Edwards WD. Pathology of radiation-induced heart disease: a surgical and autopsy study of 27 cases. Hum Pathol 1996;27:766–73.
27. Rullan E, Sigal LH. Rheumatic fever. Curr Rheumatol Rep 2001;3:445–52.
28. Cunningham MW. Autoimmunity and molecular mimicry in the pathogenesis of post-Streptococcal heart disease. Front Biosci 2003;8:s533–45.
29. Cunningham MW. T cell mimicry in inflammatory heart disease. Mol Immunol 2004;40:1121–7.
30. Hilario MO, Terreri MT. Rheumatic fever and post-streptococcal arthritis. Best Pract Res Clin Rheumatol 2002;16:481–94.

31. Dare AJ, Harrity PJ, Tazelaar HD, et al. Evaluation of surgically excised mitral valves: revised recommendations based on changing operative procedures in the 1990s. Hum Pathol 1993;24:1286–93.

32. Wilkins GT, Weyman AE, Abascal VM, et al. Percutaneous balloon dilatation of the mitral valve: an analysis of echocardiographic variables related to outcome and the mechanism of dilatation. Br Heart J 1988;60:299–308.

33. Anwar AM, Attia WM, Nosir YF, et al. Validation of a new score for the assessment of mitral stenosis using real-time three-dimensional echocardiography. J Am Soc Echocardiogr 2010;23:13–22.

34. Hauck AJ, Edwards WD, Danielson GK, et al. Mitral and aortic valve disease associated with ergotamine therapy for migraine. Arch Pathol Lab Med 1990; 114:62–4.

35. Redfield MM, Nicholson WJ, Edwards WD, et al. Valve disease associated with ergot alkaloid use: echocardiographic and pathologic correlations. Ann Intern Med 1992;117:50–2.

36. van der Bel-Kahn J, Becker AE. The surgical pathology of rheumatic and floppy mitral valves. Distinctive morphologic features upon gross examination. Am J Surg Pathol 1986;10:282–92.

37. Waller BF, Morrow AG, Maron BJ, et al. Etiology of clinically isolated, severe, chronic, pure mitral regurgitation: analysis of 97 patients over 30 years of age having mitral valve replacement. Am Heart J 1982; 104:276–88.

38. Edwards JE. Floppy mitral valve syndrome. Cardiovasc Clin 1988;18:249–71.

39. Mesana T, Ibrahim M, Hynes M. A technique for annular plication to facilitate sliding plasty after extensive mitral valve posterior leaflet resection. Ann Thorac Surg 2005;79:720–2.

40. Connolly HM, Crary JL, McGoon MD, et al. Valvular heart disease associated with fenfluramine-phentermine. N Engl J Med 1997;337:581–8.

41. Sachdev M, Miller WC, Ryan T, et al. Effect of fenfluramine-derivative diet pills on cardiac valves: a meta-analysis of observational studies. Am Heart J 2002;144:1065–73.

42. Steffee CH, Singh HK, Chitwood WR. Histologic changes in three explanted native cardiac valves following use of fenfluramines. Cardiovasc Pathol 1999;8:245–53.

43. Volmar KE, Hutchins GM. Aortic and mitral fenfluramine-phentermine valvulopathy in 64 patients treated with anorectic agents. Arch Pathol Lab Med 2001;125:1555–61.

44. Pritchett AM, Morrison JF, Edwards WD, et al. Valvular heart disease in patients taking pergolide. Mayo Clin Proc 2002;77:1280–6.

45. Hong ZG, Smith AJ, Archer SL, et al. Pergolide is an inhibitor of voltage-gated potassium channels, including Kv1.5, and causes pulmonary vasoconstriction. Circulation 2005;112:1494–9.

46. Grande-Allen KJ, Griffin BP, Calabro A, et al. Myxomatous mitral valve chordae. II: selective elevation of glycosaminoglycan content. J Heart Valve Dis 2001;10:325–32.

47. Barber JE, Ratliff NB, Cosgrove DM III, et al. Myxomatous mitral valve chordae. I: mechanical properties. J Heart Valve Dis 2001;10:320–4.

48. Carpentier AF, Pellerin M, Fuzellier JF, et al. Extensive calcification of the mitral valve anulus: pathology and surgical management. J Thorac Cardiovasc Surg 1996;111:718–29.

49. Sia YT, Dulay D, Burwash IG, et al. Mobile ventricular thrombus arising from the mitral annulus in patients with dense mitral annular calcification. Eur J Echocardiogr 2010;2:198–201.

50. Waller BF, Howard J, Fess S. Pathology of tricuspid valve stenosis and pure tricuspid regurgitation– Part I. Clin Cardiol 1995;18:97–102.

51. Waller BF, Howard J, Fess S. Pathology of tricuspid valve stenosis and pure tricuspid regurgitation– Part II. Clin Cardiol 1995;18:167–74.

52. Banning AP, Durrani A, Pillai R. Rupture of the atrial septum and tricuspid valve after blunt chest trauma. Ann Thorac Surg 1997;64:240–2.

53. Chares M, Lamm P, Leischik R, et al. Highly acute course of ruptured papillary muscle of the tricuspid valve in a case of blunt chest trauma. Thorac Cardiovasc Surg 1993;41:325–7.

54. Kleikamp G, Schnepper U, Kortke H, et al. Tricuspid valve regurgitation following blunt thoracic trauma. Chest 1992;102:1294–6.

55. Choi JS, Kim EJ. Simultaneous rupture of the mitral and tricuspid valves with left ventricular rupture caused by blunt trauma. Ann Thorac Surg 2008;86:1371–3.

56. Mielniczuk L, Haddad H, Davies RA, et al. Tricuspid valve chordal tissue in endomyocardial biopsy specimens of patients with significant tricuspid regurgitation. J Heart Lung Transplant 2005;24:1586–90.

57. Braverman AC, Coplen SE, Mudge GH, et al. Ruptured chordae tendineae of the tricuspid valve as a complication of endomyocardial biopsy in heart transplant patients. Am J Cardiol 1990;66:111–3.

58. Ohmori T, Iwakawa K, Matsumoto Y, et al. A fatal case of fungal endocarditis of the tricuspid valve associated with long-term venous catheterization and treatment with antibiotics in a patient with a history of alcohol abuse. Mycopathologia 1997; 139:123–8.

59. Panidis IP, Kotler MN, Mintz GS, et al. Clinical and echocardiographic correlations in right heart endocarditis. Int J Cardiol 1984;6:17–34.

60. Van Der Westhuizen NG, Rose AG. Right-sided valvular infective endocarditis: a clinicopathological study of 29 patients. S Afr Med J 1987;71:25–7.

61. Barbara DW, Edwards WD, Connolly HM, et al. Surgical pathology of 104 tricuspid valves (2000-2005) with classic right-sided Ebstein's malformation. Cardiovasc Pathol 2008;17:166–71.

62. Simula DV, Edwards WD, Tazelaar HD, et al. Surgical pathology of carcinoid heart disease: a study of 139 valves from 75 patients spanning 20 years. Mayo Clin Proc 2002;77:139–47.

63. Xu J, Jian B, Chu R, et al. Serotonin mechanisms in heart valve disease II: the 5-HT2 receptor and its signaling pathway in aortic valve interstitial cells. Am J Pathol 2002;161:2209–18.

64. Jian B, Xu J, Connolly J, et al. Serotonin mechanisms in heart valve disease I: serotonin-induced up-regulation of transforming growth factor-{beta}1 via G-protein signal transduction in aortic valve interstitial cells. Am J Pathol 2002;161:2111–21.

65. Walker GA, Masters KS, Shah DN, et al. Valvular myofibroblast activation by transforming growth factor-beta: implications for pathological extracellular matrix remodeling in heart valve disease. Circ Res 2004;95:253–60.

66. Shworak NW. Angiogenic modulators in valve development and disease:does valvular disease recapitulate developmental signaling pathways? Curr Opin Cardiol 2004;19:140–6.

67. Anderson KR, Zuberbuhler JR, Anderson RH, et al. Morphologic spectrum of Ebstein's anomaly of the heart: a review. Mayo Clin Proc 1979;54:174–80.

68. Ho HH, Min JK, Lin F, et al. Calcified amorphous tumor of the heart. Circulation 2008;117:E171–2.

69. Waller BF, Howard J, Fess S. Pathology of pulmonic valve stenosis and pure regurgitation. Clin Cardiol 1995;18:45–50.

70. Baddour LM, Bettmann MA, Bolger AF, et al. Non-valvular cardiovascular device-related infections. Circulation 2003;108:2015–31.

71. Arber N, Pras E, Copperman Y, et al. Pacemaker endocarditis. Report of 44 cases and review of the literature. Medicine 1994;73:299–305.

72. Rubinstein E, Lang R. Fungal endocarditis. Eur Heart J 1995;16(Suppl B):84–9.

73. Durack DT. Prevention of infective endocarditis. N Engl J Med 1995;332:38–44.

74. Atkinson JB, Virmani R. Infective endocarditis: changing trends and general approach for examination. Hum Pathol 1987;18:603–8.

75. Fernicola DJ, Roberts WC. Clinicopathologic features of active infective endocarditis isolated to the native mitral valve. Am J Cardiol 1993;71:1186–97.

76. Walsh TJ, Hutchins GM, Bulkley BH, et al. Fungal infections of the heart: analysis of 51 autopsy cases. Am J Cardiol 1980;45:357–66.

77. Isotalo PA, Chan KL, Rubens F, et al. Prosthetic valve fungal endocarditis due to histoplasmosis. Can J Cardiol 2001;17:297–303.

78. Atkinson JB, Connor DH, Robinowitz M, et al. Cardiac fungal infections: review of autopsy findings in 60 patients. Hum Pathol 1984;15:935–42.

79. Muehrcke DD. Fungal prosthetic valve endocarditis. Semin Thorac Cardiovasc Surg 1995;7:20–4.

80. Ellis M. Fungal endocarditis. J Infect 1997;35:99–103.

PRACTICAL APPROACH TO THE EVALUATION OF PROSTHETIC MECHANICAL AND TISSUE REPLACEMENT HEART VALVES

Paul A. VanderLaan, MD, PhD*, Robert F. Padera, MD, PhD,
Fredrick J. Schoen, MD, PhD

KEYWORDS

- Substitute heart valve • Bioprosthetic • Mechanical • Complication • Medical device

ABSTRACT

Mechanical and bioprosthetic substitute heart valves have dramatically improved life expectancy and quality of life in patients with valvular heart disease. Complications of substitute heart valves are a relatively infrequent occurrence, and principally due to thrombosis, infection, or structural/mechanical failure. It is important to accurately identify and systematically evaluate prosthetic heart valves when encountered as surgical pathology specimens or in the autopsy setting.

OVERVIEW OF PROSTHETIC HEART VALVES

In the half-century since the first successful cardiac valve replacement surgeries, millions of patients have benefited from this life saving procedure. It is estimated that approximately 90,000 valve replacements are performed yearly in the United States, with worldwide numbers near 300,000.[1] Patients with heart valve dysfunction due to stenosis or regurgitation gain significant survival and quality-of-life improvements with valve replacement.

There have been numerous iterations of valve designs over the years, but prosthetic valves can be broadly classified as either mechanical or tissue. Most tissue valve replacements are *bioprosthetic*, a term that describes tissue that is chemically treated before implantation. Both mechanical and tissue valves respond passively to pressure gradients through the cardiac cycle and facilitate unidirectional blood flow through the heart. Mechanical valves are composed of synthetic biomaterials that use a rigid but mobile occluder; designs have included caged ball, caged disc, tilting disc, or bileaflet tilting disc configurations (bileaflet tilting disc designs are most commonly used today). Bioprosthetic valves on the other hand are composed of flexible biologic materials, usually either porcine aortic valve or bovine pericardial tissue (pre-fixed in glutaraldehyde), and have a trileaflet structure that mimics that of native semilunar valves.[2–4]

Although numerous factors are taken into account in the clinical decision of whether to implant a mechanical, bioprosthetic or other tissue valve, the primary consideration often weighs the risk of lifelong anticoagulant therapy and the consequent risk of anticoagulation-related hemorrhage necessitated by mechanical valves versus

Disclosures: P.A.V. has nothing to disclose. R.F.P. has been a consultant to the following valve developers and manufacturers in the past five years: Medtronic, St. Jude Medical, Sadra/Boston Scientific, Direct Flow Medical, Mitral Solutions, and Sorin. F.J.S. has been a consultant to the following valve developers and manufacturers in the past five years: Celxcel, Edwards Lifesciences, Medtronic, P-R-Square, St. Jude Medical, Sadra/Boston Scientific, Direct Flow Medical, Mitral Solutions, Sulzer Carbomedics and Sorin.
Department of Pathology, Brigham and Women's Hospital, Harvard Medical School, 75 Francis Street, Boston, MA 02115, USA
* Corresponding author.
E-mail address: pvanderlaan@partners.org

Surgical Pathology 5 (2012) 353–369
doi:10.1016/j.path.2012.03.002

surgpath.theclinics.com

Key Features
CAUSES OF FAILURE AND OTHER KEY PATHOLOGIC FEATURES TO BE ASSESSED IN SUBSTITUTE HEART VALVES

Gross Examination	Identification of valve type, model, and manufacturer
	Thrombus
	Vegetation
	Calcification (pannus and/or cusps)
	Cusp or occluder mobility
	[a]Cusp fenestrations/tears
	[a]Cusp abrasion
	[a]Cusp stretching
	[a]Strut orientation/distortion and cuspal attachments
	Mechanical dysfunction, wear, or fracture
	Tissue overgrowth (pannus formation)
	Extrinsic interference or damage
	Suture or tissue entrapment
	[a]Root dilation (stentless tissue valve)
	Abnormality of anatomic orientation (autopsy)
	Paravalvular leak (autopsy)
	Device serial number (may be useful in reporting a product failure to the manufacturer and/or regulatory agency)
Radiography	Identification of valve type, model, and manufacturer (may be helpful)
	[a]Calcification: degree, location
	Ring/stent/poppet abnormalities
Histology	[a]Cusp architecture, integrity, and delamination
	Thrombus formation
	Vegetation: acute inflammation, microorganisms (Gram, MSS stains)
	[a]Calcification
	Tissue overgrowth (pannus formation)
	Endothelialization (sewing cuff and tissue)
	[a]Cusp fluid insudation and hematoma
	Host reaction (sewing cuff and cusps: chronic inflammation, foreign body giant cell reaction)

[a] For tissue valves/bioprostheses only.

the significantly higher rate of structural valve deterioration for bioprosthetic valves.[1,4] Calcific or non-calcific structural failure necessitating re-operation within 10 to 15 years is much more common in recipients of bioprosthetic valves.[5,6] As such, mechanical valves are usually recommended for younger patients to obviate the need for multiple valve replacement re-operations over their lifetime.[7] Overall, mechanical and bioprosthetic valves are implanted in roughly equal proportions, although the latter type has increasingly been used in recent years.[8]

This chapter will provide the reader with an up-to-date overview and approach to the analysis of different prosthetic valves that may be encountered as surgical pathology or autopsy specimens (and potentially in a research setting). Identification of the specific prosthetic valve type and the common pathologic complications and structural features to be evaluated will be highlighted. Finally, a discussion of other valve prostheses and substitutions less commonly encountered and in development or early clinical application will be presented.

APPROACH TO EVALUATION OF THE PROSTHETIC HEART VALVE

- Obtain proper clinical history.
- Perform gross evaluation.
- Identify prosthesis manufacturer and model.
- Photograph specimen.
- Obtain specimen radiograph where necessary.
- Record device serial number (if indicated).
- Submit histologic sections of bioprosthetic valve cusps (decalcify as necessary).
- Submit tissue adherent to the sewing ring from both mechanical and bioprosthetic valves.
- Examine for evidence of active infection.
- Submit valvular vegetations, thrombi, or tissue overgrowth with gram or silver stains useful for the identification of infective endocarditis.

Pathologists typically encounter prosthetic heart valves for evaluation as either a surgical reoperation specimen or at autopsy. In both instances, a proper clinical history is crucial before the subsequent assessment of the prosthetic valve, placing into context any observations made by the pathologist. With this information, gross evaluation of the valve begins with the proper identification of the mechanical prosthesis, bioprosthetic valve, or other tissue valve. Reviewing the original clinical and operative notes, as well as consultation with the surgeon sometimes is useful for the identification of the manufacturer and model of the explanted valve prosthesis, though this information is not always readily available. Importantly, since patients may live many decades following valve replacement, pathologists may encounter valves no longer used. In such instances, the reader is directed to additional published resources for a more detailed discussion and comprehensive set of images to aid in the identification of specific prosthetic valves.[3,9–12]

The specimen should be photographed before extensive manipulation, and radiographs may prove helpful for identification and in evaluating the degree of calcification for bioprosthetic valves.[13] In general, attention should be paid to the three main valve components:

1. Moveable part(s)
2. Superstructure that guides the movement of and/or anchors the mobile occluder(s) or tissue
3. Sewing cuff.

When necessary for reporting serious device-related failure to the FDA and/or the manufacturer, one should record the unique device serial number, usually placed by the manufacturer under the sewing ring at the valve base. As outlined in a recent consensus statement by the Society for Cardiovascular Pathology and the Association for European Cardiovascular Pathology[14] and elsewhere,[3,15] the gross assessment of the valve should include:

1. measurement of the sewing ring external diameter
2. extent of tissue overgrowth
3. irregularities (tears or perforations) or structural defects (abrasions or cracks) of the valve cusps
4. presence of calcification
5. presence and location of thrombi or vegetations
6. evaluation of the range of movement and closure of the valve cusps.

Histologic sections should be submitted of the bioprosthetic valve cusps, taken perpendicular to the sewing ring. Decalcification may be necessary when calcific deposits are present. Additionally, tissue adherent to the sewing ring should be submitted from both mechanical and bioprosthetic valves, which often demonstrates blood insudation, fibrosis, chronic inflammation, and foreign body giant cell reaction to polarizable sewing cuff material. The degree of healing and pathologic appearance of the tissue associated with a sewing cuff is highly variable among patients, often despite long implant times. Close examination for evidence of active infection should be performed. Additionally, any valvular vegetations, thrombi, or tissue overgrowth should be submitted, with gram or silver stains useful for the identification of infective endocarditis. Finally, care should be taken not to over-interpret changes to the valve introduced during the surgical procedure to remove it; communication with the surgeon or reference to the operative note can be helpful in such instances.

COMMON TYPES OF PROSTHETIC HEART VALVES

MECHANICAL VALVES

Of the numerous iterations on the mechanical heart valve design over the past 50 years, the vast majority can be classified into one of four main categories: caged ball, caged disc, tilting disc, and bileaflet tilting disc valves (**Figs. 1** and **2**).[3,10–12] The caged ball design (see **Fig. 1A**) relies on a freely movable ball occluder that is held in place by a wire cage attached to the orifice ring. This valve design has been in use longer than any other, first introduced in the early 1960s, though is not available today. The caged disc valve design (see **Fig. 1B**) is similar in principle to the caged ball, but has a lower profile due to the flat disc occluder; this design was popular in the

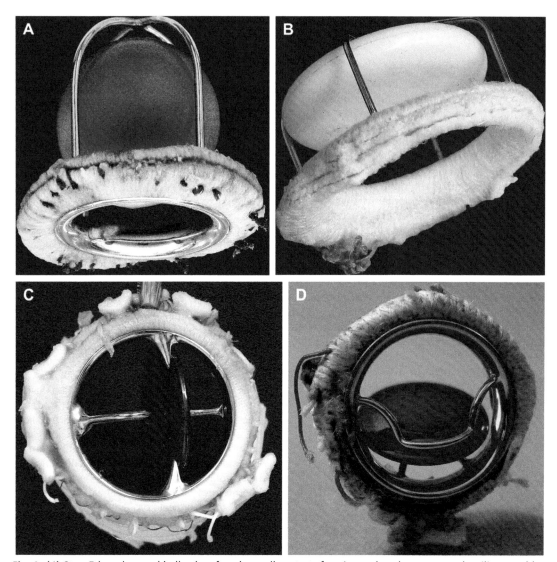

Fig. 1. (*A*) Starr-Edwards caged ball valve: four bare alloy struts forming a closed cage around a silicone rubber (Silastic) poppet with a knitted Teflon sewing ring. This mitral valve prosthesis was removed after 48 years implantation for paravalvular leak. (*B*) Harken caged disc valve, with four bare alloy struts forming a closed cage around a plastic disc with a cloth-covered sewing ring. (*C*) Medtronic-Hall single leaflet tilting disc valve: a pyrolytic carbon poppet with an opening angle of 70–75° in a titanium housing with a knitted Teflon sewing ring. (*D*) Bjork-Shiley single leaflet tilting disc valve: a flat pyrolytic carbon poppet with central depression, opening angle of 60°, with dual alloy struts (large inflow and small outflow) and Teflon sewing ring.

1960s, but is not used today. The tilting disc valve (see **Fig. 1**C and D) was first introduced in approximately 1970 with the aim to lessen the obstruction to blood flow through the valve that characterized the caged ball and caged disc designs. These valves have a single circular pyrolytic carbon disc that opens and closes by pivoting about metal struts that also hold the disc in place. The most recent class of mechanical valve is the bileaflet tilting-disc design (see **Fig. 2**). Accounting for the vast majority of mechanical valves implanted today, these valves have two semicircular valve

leaflets composed of pyrolytic carbon, which pivot on hinges at the periphery.

BIOPROSTHETIC VALVES

Structurally and functionally, bioprosthetic tissue valves more closely resemble native valves than do mechanical valves. Attached to the fabric covered sewing cuff are struts on which the valve tissue is mounted. Bioprosthetic valve tissue is generally derived from either bovine pericardium or porcine aortic valve (**Figs. 3** and **4**). Recipients of

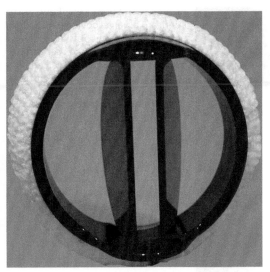

Fig. 2. St. Jude Medical bileaflet tilting disc valve: the most commonly implanted mechanical valve. Bileaflet pyrolytic carbon discs encased in a pyrolytic carbon housing with a woven Teflon sewing ring.

bioprosthetic valves (or homograft/autograft valves, discussed later) do not require immunosuppressive therapy; these heterograft/xenograft materials are glutaraldehyde fixed and often treated with anti-mineralization agents.[6,9] The microscopic architecture of these two bioprosthetic valve types is different; porcine aortic valves retain the tri-layered orientation of the fibrosa, spongiosa, and ventricularis layers with natural cuspal edges and attachments, whereas bovine pericardium demonstrates a more homogeneous laminated fibrous tissue structure with cuspal edges and attachments fabricated by the manufacturer.[3]

Stented bioprosthetic valves have a smaller effective transvalvular orifice area than native valves due to the space occupied by the mounting struts, which can become problematic when the intended recipient has a small native aortic or pulmonic valve annulus. In such situations, a stentless bioprosthetic valve is sometimes used. These valves are comprised of porcine aortic valve and aortic root, with or without the coronary ostia and are not mounted on frame (**Fig. 5**).[16,17]

PROSTHETIC HEART VALVE COMPLICATIONS

Evaluation of a prosthetic valve on the surgical pathology cutting bench more often than not implies dysfunction or failure. Even in appropriately managed patients, the overall annual incidence of prosthetic valve complications is around 3 to 4%.[5,18–20] An overview of the most common prosthetic valve complications is presented here with selected examples provided. For a more in-depth discussion of the structure and function of mechanical and tissue valves and the specific modes of prosthetic valve failure with illustrative examples, the reader is directed to a number of comprehensive resources.[3,21–23]

THROMBOEMBOLIC COMPLICATIONS

Thrombosis is a potential problem for patients with both mechanical and bioprosthetic valves. Mechanical valves are more vulnerable to thrombotic complications, due to the introduction of foreign biomaterial, higher shear stress, disturbed flow, and mechanical trauma of blood elements. These factors lead to a localized procoagulant environment, necessitating lifelong systemic anticoagulation to prevent thrombosis in recipients of mechanical valves.

Thromboembolism as a complication of mechanical heart valves is a constant risk, especially in the situation where anticoagulation is suboptimal. Over time this risk has decreased, owing to improved mechanical valve design and better titration of anticoagulation management.[24] The risk of bioprosthetic valve thrombosis is less, and most often occurs in the first few months following implantation before complete endothelialization of the sewing cuff.[22] There is a higher risk of thrombotic complications for those infrequent instances when a mechanical or bioprosthetic valve is placed in the tricuspid position, likely due to decreased flow velocity through right sided chambers.[25]

Thrombotic deposits generally occur on the outflow aspects of valves (**Figs. 6** and **7**). Mechanical valve thrombosis involving the hinge regions can lead to fixation of the disk in an open position, resulting in valvular insufficiency.[26] Extensive thrombus formation can also occlude the valve orifice, causing functional stenosis with a resultant pressure gradient. Care must be taken (especially in the autopsy setting) to differentiate postmortem clot about the valve from true prosthesis thrombosis; the former typically are ill formed and only loosely adherent to the valve surface. Because of the lack of adjacent vascularized tissue in valve prostheses, thrombus organization is impaired, making dating of a thrombus difficult on histologic evaluation (ie, thrombosis may have been present for a longer time than suggested histologically).[2]

INFECTIOUS COMPLICATIONS

Prosthetic valve infective endocarditis (PVE) is an infrequent complication with a high mortality.

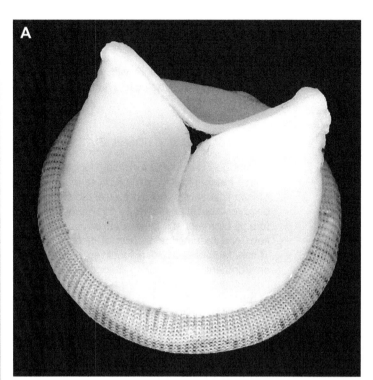

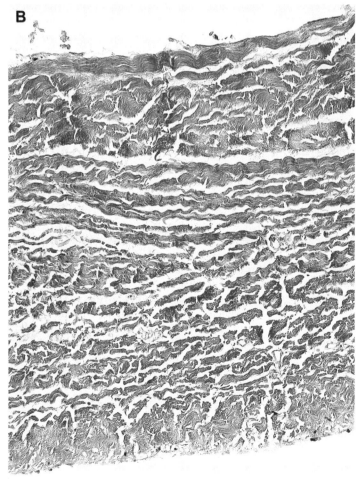

Fig. 3. (A) Sorin Mitroflow aortic pericardial valve: bovine pericardium mounted on the outside of three struts. (B) Histologic section of a bovine pericardial valve, demonstrating largely decellularized tissue with uniform collagen bundles and interstitial fibroelastosis (H&E stain, 200x original magnification).

Fig. 4. (*A*) Hancock (Medtronic) stented porcine aortic valve. (*B*) Histologic section of a porcine aortic valve, demonstrating the largely decellularized trilayered normal valvular architecture: the collagen dense fibrosa (f), the loose connective mucopolysaccharide spongiosa (s), and elastin-rich ventricularis (v) can be appreciated from superior to inferior (H&E stain, 100x original magnification).

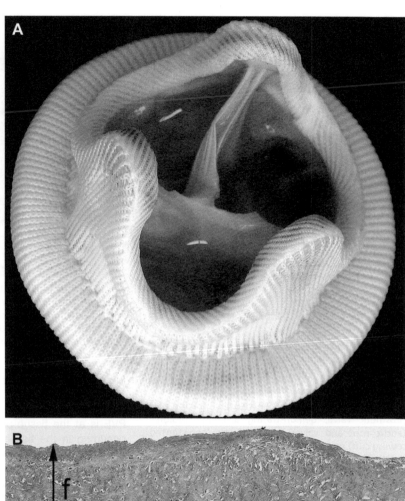

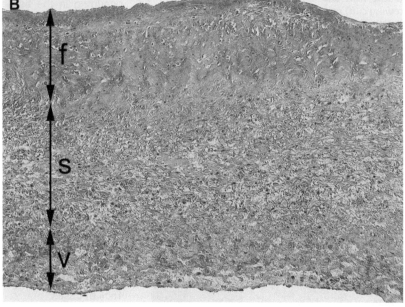

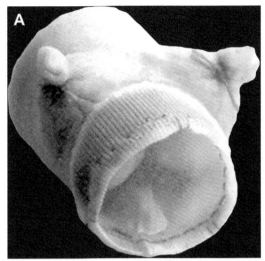

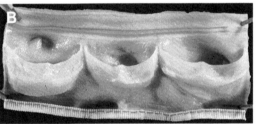

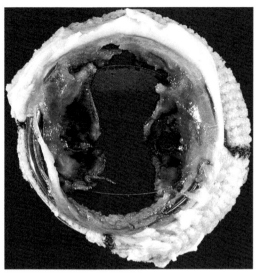

Fig. 7. St. Jude Medical bileaflet tilting disc valve with extensive thrombosis involving the inflow (shown) and outflow surfaces, fixing the valve in an open position. Note the marked adherence to the device and signs of early organization near the sewing ring.

Fig. 5. (*A*) Medtronic Freestyle stentless porcine bioprosthetic valve, demonstrating a hybrid biologic (aortic root and valves) and synthetic (non-stented sewing cuff) prosthesis. (*B*) Prosthesis opened longitudinally to reveal the three native valve cusps with preserved coronary ostia.

Mechanical and bioprosthetic valves are affected at a similar rate.

For mechanical valves, the most common site of PVE is at the tissue-prosthesis junction, usually occurring in the tissue immediately adjacent to the sewing cuff. Infection at the sewing ring can lead to ring abscess formation, prosthesis dehiscence, paravalvular leak, heart block, and septic embolization.[2] Although bioprosthetic PVE also often involves the sewing ring, involvement of the valve cusps *per se* is commonly encountered, which can lead to cuspal thickening, stiffening or perforation with valvular insufficiency, and often calcification (**Fig. 8**).

The infectious agent in PVE is bacterial in the vast majority of cases, most commonly caused by *Staphylococcus aureus*, coagulase-negative *Staphylococcus*, *Streptococcus viridans*, and *Enterococci*.[27] Fungal infection is rare (less than 5% of cases), though more common in PVE than in native valve endocarditis.[28] Gram and silver/fungal stains should be performed on infected materials to help identify the infectious agent, as blood culture results are negative in approximately 15% of cases.[2]

STRUCTURAL/MECHANICAL COMPLICATIONS

Although the lifelong anticoagulation therapy needed with mechanical valves is usually obviated with bioprosthetic valves, tissue degeneration and calcification are major issues limiting

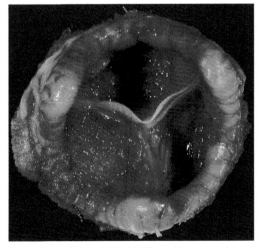

Fig. 6. Biocor (St. Jude Medical) porcine stented aortic valve prosthesis with extensive cuspal thrombosis affecting the outflow surfaces. No histologic evidence of infection was identified.

Fig. 8. (*A*) Carpentier-Edwards bovine pericardial bioprosthetic valve with infective endocarditis; large vegetation present on the outflow surface at the sewing ring-valve interface. (*B*) Histologic examination revealed a neutrophil-rich thrombus (H&E, original magnification 400x); abundant bacteria can be seen within the tissue on the H&E stained section.

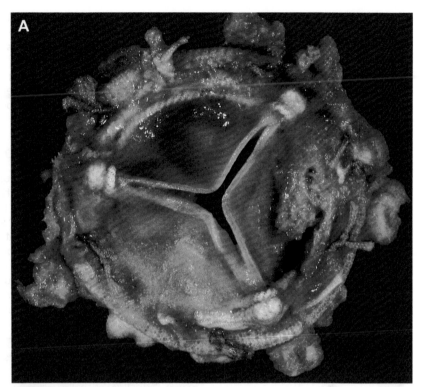

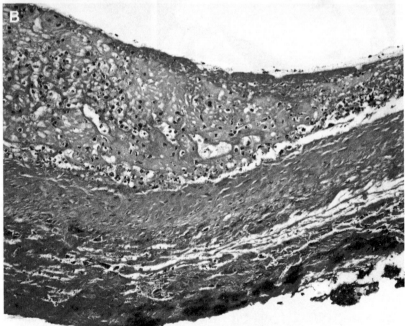

long-term success of bioprostheses in many patients. These complications are gradual and progressive in nature, eventually necessitating a repeat operative valve replacement. Approximately a quarter of bioprosthetic valves fail within 10 years of implantation, and around 50% experience dysfunction due to tissue degeneration by 15 years post-implantation.[5,19,22] Structural valve deterioration tends to begin earlier with porcine aortic valves as compared with bovine pericardial valves.[7] Furthermore, bioprosthetic valves implanted in younger individuals and patients with type II diabetes or the metabolic syndrome tend to have an increased rate and rapidity of bioprosthetic structural valve degeneration.[6,22,29,30] Gross examination of such bioprosthetic valves can demonstrate nodular calcification of the valve cusps and cuspal tears (Figs. 9 and 10). Radiographs of the explanted bioprosthetic valve can provide a means of semiquantitative assessment of calcific burden.[13]

In general, the structural failure or material fracture of mechanical valves in clinical use today is exceedingly low, due to strenuous pre-clinical device testing and the use of extremely durable biomaterials (eg, titanium, pyrolytic carbon). The few reported device failures mainly include fracture of a valve strut due to metal fatigue or fracture of the carbon disk, leading to fatal acute valvular insufficiency and embolization of valve components.[2,31,32] Pathological examination of

the explanted mechanical valve (or mechanical valves in the autopsy setting) should include a search for any cracks, areas of wear, or structural defects. However, as the surgeon is clearly more concerned with a safe and efficient operation than a pristine specimen, artifactual trauma to the specimen can occur inadvertently at the time of removal.

NON-STRUCTURAL COMPLICATIONS

Prosthetic valve failure can also occur as a result of defective healing at the prosthesis-tissue interface, resulting in a paravalvular leak. Most commonly, paravalvular leaks result from infection (which may be healed at the time of examination), a defect in suture knot placement or tying, or from degeneration (calcific or myxomatous) of the tissue adjacent to the suture ring.[2] In some cases the cause of a paravalvular leak may not be apparent. Elevated transvalvular pressures due

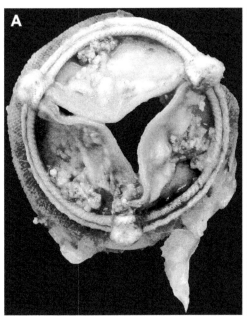

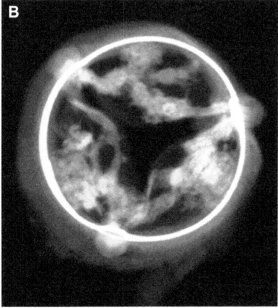

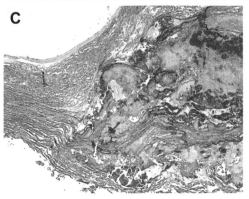

Fig. 9. (A) Carpentier-Edwards bovine pericardial bioprosthetic valve demonstrating characteristic nodular calcium deposits resulting in cuspal stiffness and valvular stenosis. (B) Specimen radiograph demonstrating an intact ring with a 3+ (out of 4) grade calcification score. (C) Histologic section (following decalcification) demonstrates the large amorphous areas of calcific degeneration with paucity of inflammatory cells or evidence of osseous metaplasia, features which are frequently seen in native valves undergoing calcific degeneration.

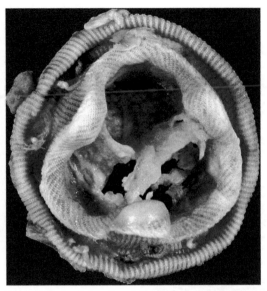

Fig. 10. Hancock (Medtronic) porcine aortic valve bioprosthesis demonstrating cuspal calcific degeneration (2+ out of 4 by radiograph) and severe microscopic degeneration, with grossly apparent cuspal tears, resulting in valvular insufficiency.

to patient-prosthetic mismatch (ie, when the intrinsic obstruction of the prosthesis is limiting or the valve implanted is too small) are seen in 20 to 70% of aortic valve prostheses.[33] In these cases, the valve received on the surgical bench may very well appear normal. Excessive healing, manifest as exuberant pannus overgrowth may interfere with the movement of the occluder or

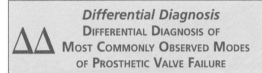

Differential Diagnosis
DIFFERENTIAL DIAGNOSIS OF MOST COMMONLY OBSERVED MODES OF PROSTHETIC VALVE FAILURE

- Thrombosis (Mechanical > Bioprosthetic)
- Infection
- Leaflet/cuspal tissue deterioration (Bioprosthetic only)
- Structural/mechanical failure
- Tissue pannus overgrowth
- Entrapped suture or foreign material
- Paravalvular leak (seen by the pathologist at autopsy)

cause stiffening of valve cusps, leading to functional regurgitation or stenosis (**Figs. 11 and 12**). Loose suture ends can get caught in the valve orifice of mechanical valves, thereby preventing full closure, or can become stiff over time and puncture bioprosthetic valve cusps.[3] An immunologic-mediated inflammatory reaction to foreign tissues in xenograft valves has been proposed but not confirmed as a mode of failure.[34] Clinically relevant hemolysis can be seen in the setting of a prosthetic valve and is usually associated with either structural deterioration or paravalvular leak.[35] Coronary ostial occlusion or stenosis is an uncommon complication encountered in surgical replacement of the aortic valve.[36]

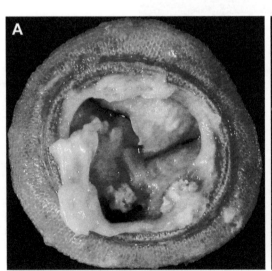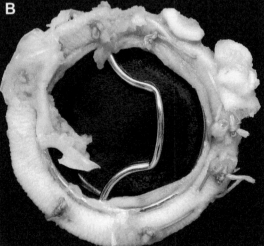

Fig. 11. (*A*) Carpentier-Edwards bovine pericardial bioprosthesis with significant calcification (4+ out of 4 by radiograph) and focal pannus overgrowth. (*B*) Bjork-Shiley single leaflet tilting disc valve with focal pannus overgrowth of the inflow surface that became trapped in the valve orifice, preventing full closure of the valve poppet.

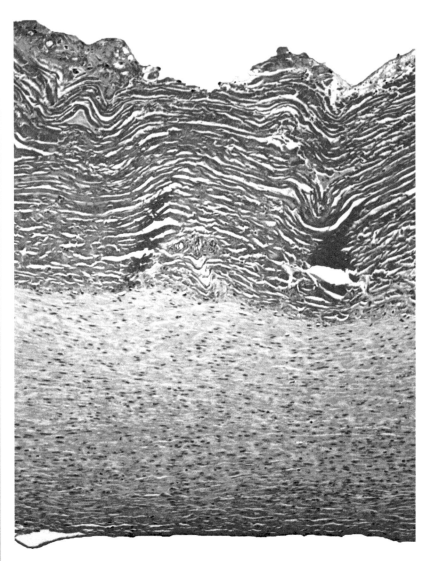

Fig. 12. Histologic example of thick pannus overgrowth of a bovine pericardial bioprosthetic valve. Note the bland cellularity of the tissue pannus (*bottom*) in contrast to the largely decellularized pericardial valve leaflet (*top*), without evidence of acute inflammation or structural degeneration.

OTHER HEART VALVES AND FUTURE CONSIDERATIONS

HOMOGRAFT AND AUTOGRAFT TISSUE VALVES

Other tissue valve replacements used clinically include homograft (allograft) valves, which are native valves typically derived from deceased humans or less often from explant hearts, and autograft valves (the patient's own valve surgically moved to a new position). Cadaveric allograft valves demonstrate excellent hemodynamics, low thrombogenicity without necessitating chronic anticoagulation or immunosuppression, and a low infection rate.[3] Allograft valves are generally chemically sterilized and cryopreserved following harvest, allowing for long-term storage or banking.

As with bioprosthetic valves, structural deterioration is the most common cause of allograft valve failure, with 50 to 90% valve survival in the 10- to 15-year window following transplant.[3] In contrast to autograft valves discussed below (which are neither cryopreserved nor have significant ischemic times), allograft valves do not generally have viable cells at the time of implantation.[37] Failure of these devitalized allograft valves is characterized by calcification with associated cuspal perforation, rupture, or tearing when implanted on the left side, whereas stenosis with or without calcification of the valve and supporting transplanted vascular wall typifies right-sided implants.[3,37]

First reported in 1967, the replacement of a dysfunctional aortic valve by the patient's own pulmonic valve (autograft) is known as the Ross procedure.[38] This procedure is typically performed on younger or middle age patients. In the traditional Ross procedure, the aortic valve is replaced by the patient's own viable and hemodynamically sound pulmonic valve, which in turn is replaced most typically with a devitalized allograft valve.[39]

The long-term pathologic follow-up for patients undergoing the Ross procedure is still accumulating, though around 10% of patients develop pulmonic autograft regurgitation and/or progressive aortic root dilation within 10 to 15 years, necessitating reoperation.[3,40] Histologic evaluation of the pulmonary valve autograft of such specimens reveals viable valve cusps, fibrous hyperplasia of the ventricularis layer and variable scarring of the transplanted arterial wall.[41,42] In cases of dilation of the neoaortic root leading to regurgitation and occasionally aneurysm with dissection, histologic features include intimal thickening, medial scarring, elastin fragmentation, and adventitial fibrosis.[42,43]

TRANSCATHETER AORTIC VALVE IMPLANTATION

The high mortality associated with untreated aortic stenosis, especially in elderly patients who otherwise could not tolerate open heart surgery, has led to the increasing use of minimally invasive transcatheter delivery of bioprosthetic valves.[44] Transcatheter aortic valve implantation (TAVI) is a relatively new procedure, only first performed in 2002.[45] Clinical experience with this minimally invasive procedure is growing rapidly, with over 40,000 TAVI procedures performed worldwide to date.[46] At the time of writing, there are two transcatheter aortic-valve devices currently approved by the FDA for use in the United States: the Edwards Sapien aortic valve (Edwards Lifesciences) and the CoreValve (Medtronic), though many other models are in development.[46]

The catheter-deployed bioprosthetic aortic valves have an expandable metal stent frame, similar to traditional coronary artery stents, encasing either glutaraldehyde-pretreated bovine or porcine pericardial valve leaflets (Fig. 13); the device must be compressed to approximately 7 mm diameter to be ensheathed within a delivery catheter. The valves come in a range of expanded diameters (23 to 26 mm), enabling a good match with the target valve orifice. Importantly, in this procedure the diseased aortic valve is not removed; it is merely pushed out toward the periphery by the device. In addition to these transcatheter aortic valves, the Melody transcatheter pulmonary valve (Medtronic) is designed for use in patients with a failing right ventricular outflow tract conduit, and is composed of an expandable stent housing a segment of bovine jugular vein with its native venous valve (Fig. 14).[47] Transcatheter-deployed valves have been used

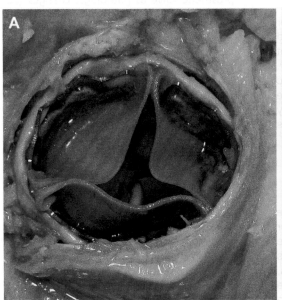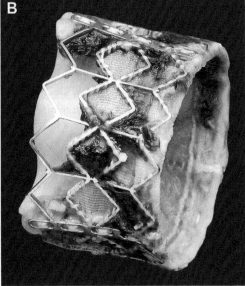

Fig. 13. (*A*) Edwards Sapien bovine pericardial transcatheter-deployed aortic valve visualized from the aortic aspect. The expandable stent frame is tightly opposed to the native aortic valve without evidence of paravalvular leak. (*B*) Lateral view of the prosthesis after removal from the aortic root. The loosely adherent blood clot is post-mortem in nature, not to be confused with true pathologic pre-mortem thrombosis.

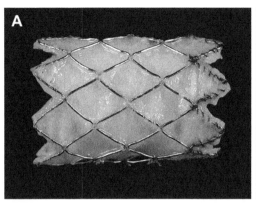
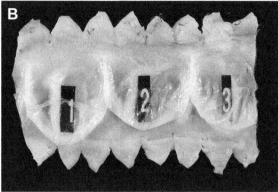

Fig. 14. (A) Melody (Medtronic) transcatheter pulmonary valve bioprosthesis, external view demonstrating the platinum-iridium stent housing. (B) Prosthesis opened to reveal the three delicate bovine jugular vein valve cusps.

in all four cardiac valve positions, and also provide the opportunity of deployment within a previously failed bioprosthetic valve. This *valve-in-valve* approach can effectively treat transvalvular regurgitation, incompetence, or stenosis, and early studies report excellent hemodynamic and functional outcomes in these patients.[48]

In addition to the procedural and peri-procedural risks, complications (both reported and theoretical) include paravalvular leak, occlusion of the coronary ostia by a valve strut during deployment, aorta-atrial fistula formation, and valve embolization.[49,50] Case reports of acute bacterial or fungal endocarditis in patients undergoing TAVI highlight the problematic nature of subsequent surgical revision or replacement in these patients initially deemed unsuitable for more invasive valve replacement surgery.[51] The data on long-term durability, specific modes of failure, and related pathologic findings of this class of bioprosthetic valves are just starting to accumulate, which should rapidly grow as increasing numbers of patients use this minimally invasive valve replacement procedure.

VALVES IN DEVELOPMENT

Although current models of mechanical and tissue valves have proven effective replacements for diseased heart valves, novel prosthetic valve designs are in development.[52] These new designs look to overcome the limitations of current models, thereby replicating the form and function of native valves without the need for lifelong anticoagulation or eventual reoperation due to structural deterioration. Although not currently in clinical use at the time of writing, pathologists may encounter these types of valves in the future.

Synthetic flexible polymer valves look to provide a design that has central flow, is more highly durable than current bioprosthetic valves, and maintain the low thrombogenicity and immunogenicity of these

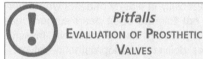

Pitfalls
EVALUATION OF PROSTHETIC VALVES

! Be sure not to over-interpret alterations induced during the surgical removal of the prosthetic valve as pathologic changes (eg, cut sutures, removal of tissue on the sewing cuff, sewing ring tears, cracks, scratches, cuspal tears, removal of material for microbiologic culture); review the operative note or consult with the surgeon.

! Do not confuse post-mortem clot (soft, deep red, poorly adherent) with pathologic pre-mortem thrombosis (firm, tan, adherent), especially in the autopsy setting; duration of thrombi may be underestimated owing to inhibited histologic organization.

! Do not confuse the histologic appearance of dystrophic calcification or foreign contaminants for bacterial infection, grossly or microscopically; identification of acute inflammation and the use of special stains may help clarify inconclusive cases. Conversely, infection may induce calcification.

! Remember to photograph and radiograph (when applicable) the specimen before extensive manipulation.

! Do not submit tissue for histologic evaluation without decalcification if gross calcific deposits are evident.

designs.[53] For these flexible leaflet valve designs, a number of polymeric materials including silicone rubber, polyurethane, polystyrene, polytetrafluoro-ethylene, and polycarbonate-urethane have been used, with valve failure in pre-clinical models often due to extrinsic calcification, thrombosis, and valve leaflet cracks.[53–55]

Work is being done to engineer a living tissue valve replacement. By seeding a patient's own valvular progenitor cells and/or endothelial cells onto a resorbable scaffold or a tissue valve that is non-viable, the promise of a immunologically silent, biologically viable valve capable of remodeling under varying physiologic stresses may be realized.[56–58] A particularly exciting possibility is that such a valve, which would have near-normal anatomy, would also have the capacity to grow with a growing patient, advantageous for children with congenital heart disease who generally have suboptimal results with existing valve replacements and who typically require multiple repeat operations as they outgrow them. Although this approach is in the early stages of development and implementation overall, favorable early outcome data have been obtained with cryopreserved, decellularized pulmonary allograft subsequently coated and seeded with autologous vascular endothelial cells.[59]

REFERENCES

1. Pibarot P, Dumesnil JG. Prosthetic heart valves: selection of the optimal prosthesis and long-term management. Circulation 2009;119:1034–48.
2. Schoen FJ. Approach to the analysis of cardiac valve prostheses as surgical pathology or autopsy specimens. Cardiovasc Pathol 1995;4:241–55.
3. Schoen FJ. Pathology of heart valve substitution with mechanical and tissue prostheses. In: Silver MD, Gotlieb AI, Schoen FJ, editors. Cardiovascular pathology. New York: Churchill Livingstone; 2001. p. 629–77.
4. Longnecker CR, Lim MJ. Prosthetic heart valves. Cardiol Clin 2011;29:229–36.
5. Hammermeister K, Sethi GK, Henderson WG, et al. Outcomes 15 years after valve replacement with a mechanical versus a bioprosthetic valve: final report of the Veterans Affairs randomized trial. J Am Coll Cardiol 2000;36:1152–8.
6. Schoen FJ, Levy RJ. Calcification of tissue heart valve substitutes: progress toward understanding and prevention. Ann Thorac Surg 2005;79:1072–80.
7. Huang G, Rahimtoola SH. Prosthetic heart valve. Circulation 2011;123:2602–5.
8. Brown JM, O'Brien SM, Wu C, et al. Isolated aortic valve replacement in North America comprising 108,687 patients in 10 years: changes in risks, valve types, and outcomes in the Society of Thoracic Surgeons National Database. J Thorac Cardiovasc Surg 2009;137:82–90.
9. Butany J, Fayet C, Ahluwalia MS, et al. Biological replacement heart valves. Identification and evaluation. Cardiovasc Pathol 2003;12:119–39.
10. Butany J, Ahluwalia MS, Munroe C, et al. Mechanical heart valve prostheses: identification and evaluation. Cardiovasc Pathol 2003;12:322–44.
11. DeWall RA, Qasim N, Carr L. Evolution of mechanical heart valves. Ann Thorac Surg 2000;69:1612–21.
12. Gott VL, Alejo DE, Cameron DE. Mechanical heart valves: 50 years of evolution. Ann Thorac Surg 2003;76:S2230–9.
13. Schoen FJ, Kujovich JL, Webb CL, et al. Chemically determined mineral content of explanted porcine aortic valve bioprostheses: correlation with radiographic assessment of calcification and clinical data. Circulation 1987;76:1061–6.
14. Stone JR, Basso C, Baandrup UT, et al. Recommendations for processing cardiovascular surgical pathology specimens: a consensus statement from the standards and definitions committee of the Society for Cardiovascular Pathology and the Association for European Cardiovascular Pathology. Cardiovasc Pathol 2012;21:2–16.
15. Butany J, Collins MJ. Analysis of prosthetic cardiac devices: a guide for the practising pathologist. J Clin Pathol 2005;58:113–24.
16. Kobayashi J. Stentless aortic valve replacement: an update. Vasc Health Risk Manag 2011;7:345–51.
17. Gulbins H, Reichenspurner H. Which patients benefit from stentless aortic valve replacement? Ann Thorac Surg 2009;88:2061–8.
18. O'Brien MF, Harrocks S, Stafford EG, et al. The homograft aortic valve: a 29-year, 99.3% follow up of 1,022 valve replacements. J Heart Valve Dis 2001;10:334–44.
19. McClure RS, Narayanasamy N, Wiegerinck E, et al. Late outcomes for aortic valve replacement with the Carpentier-Edwards pericardial bioprosthesis: up to 17-year follow-up in 1,000 patients. Ann Thorac Surg 2010;89:1410–6.
20. Oxenham H, Bloomfield P, Wheatley DJ, et al. Twenty year comparison of a Bjork-Shiley mechanical heart valve with porcine bioprostheses. Heart 2003;89:715–21.
21. Schoen FJ, Levy RJ, Piehler HR. Pathological considerations in replacement cardiac valves. Cardiovasc Pathol 1992;1:29–52.
22. Siddiqui RF, Abraham JR, Butany J. Bioprosthetic heart valves: modes of failure. Histopathology 2009;55:135–44.
23. Schoen FJ. Mechanisms of function and disease in natural and replacement heart valves. Ann Rev Path Mech Dis 2012;7:161–83.

24. Zilla P, Brink J, Human P, et al. Prosthetic heart valves: catering for the few. Biomaterials 2008;29: 385–406.

25. Kao CL, Lu MS, Chang JP, et al. Thrombotic obstruction of a mechanical prosthetic valve in tricuspid position. Tex Heart Inst J 2009;36:261–3.

26. Harris KC, Campbell AI. Images in clinical medicine. Thrombosis of a mechanical mitral valve. N Engl J Med 2011;365:e45.

27. Lee JH, Burner KD, Fealey ME, et al. Prosthetic valve endocarditis: clinicopathological correlates in 122 surgical specimens from 116 patients (1985-2004). Cardiovasc Pathol 2011;20:26–35.

28. Habib G, Thuny F, Avierinos JF. Prosthetic valve endocarditis: current approach and therapeutic options. Prog Cardiovasc Dis 2008;50:274–81.

29. Lorusso R, Gelsomino S, Lucà F, et al. Type II diabetes mellitus is associated with faster degeneration of bioprosthetic valve: results from a propensity score-matched Italian multicenter study. Circulation 2012;125:604–14.

30. Briand M, Pibarot P, Després JP, et al. Metabolic syndrome is associated with faster degeneration of bioprosthetic valves. Circulation 2006;114: I512–7.

31. Vongpatanasin W, Hillis LD, Lange RA. Prosthetic heart valves. N Engl J Med 1996;335:407–16.

32. Mosterd A, Shahin GM, van Boven WJ, et al. Images in cardiovascular medicine. Leaflet fracture of a St. Jude mechanical bileaflet valve. Circulation 2005; 111:e280–1.

33. Dumesnil JG, Pibarot P. Prosthesis-patient mismatch: an update. Curr Cardiol Rep 2011;13:250–7.

34. O'Keefe KL, Cohle SD, McNamara JE, et al. Early catastrophic stentless valve failure secondary to possible immune reaction. Ann Thorac Surg 2011; 91:1269–72.

35. Shapira Y, Vaturi M, Sagie A. Hemolysis associated with prosthetic heart valves: a review. Cardiol Rev 2009;17:121–4.

36. Turillazzi E, Di Giammarco G, Neri M, et al. Coronary ostia obstruction after replacement of aortic valve prosthesis. Diagn Pathol 2011;6:72.

37. Mitchell RN, Jonas RA, Schoen FJ. Pathology of explanted cryopreserved allograft heart valves: comparison with aortic valves from orthotopic heart transplants. J Thorac Cardiovasc Surg 1998;115: 118–27.

38. Ross DN. Replacement of aortic and mitral valves with a pulmonary autograft. Lancet 1967;2:956–8.

39. Sievers HH, Stierle U, Charitos EI, et al. Fourteen years' experience with 501 subcoronary Ross procedures: surgical details and results. J Thorac Cardiovasc Surg 2010;140:816–22.

40. Charitos EI, Stierle U, Hanke T, et al. Long-term results of 203 Young and middle-aged patients with more than 10 years of follow-up after the original subcoronary ross operation. Ann Thorac Surg 2012; 93:495–502.

41. Mookhoek A, de Heer E, Bogers AJ, et al. Pulmonary autograft valve explants show typical degeneration. J Thorac Cardiovasc Surg 2010;139:1416–9.

42. Rabkin-Aikawa E, Aikawa M, Farber M, et al. Clinical pulmonary autograft valves: pathologic evidence of adaptive remodeling in the aortic site. J Thorac Cardiovasc Surg 2004;128:552–61.

43. Schoof PH, Takkenberg JJ, van Suylen RJ, et al. Degeneration of the pulmonary autograft: an explant study. J Thorac Cardiovasc Surg 2006; 132:1426–32.

44. Faxon DP. Transcatheter aortic valve implantation: coming of age. Circulation 2011;124:e439–40.

45. Cribier A, Eltchaninoff H, Bash A, et al. Percutaneous transcatheter implantation of an aortic valve prosthesis for calcific aortic stenosis: first human case description. Circulation 2002;106:3006–8.

46. Rodés-Cabau J. Transcatheter aortic valve implantation: current and future approaches. Nat Rev Cardiol 2012;9:15–29.

47. Lurz P, Bonhoeffer P, Taylor AM. Percutaneous pulmonary valve implantation: an update. Expert Rev Cardiovasc Ther 2009;7:823–33.

48. Gurvitch R, Tay EL, Wijesinghe N, et al. Transcatheter aortic valve implantation: lessons from the learning curve of the first 270 high-risk patients. Catheter Cardiovasc Interv 2011;78:977–84.

49. Gurvitch R, Cheung A, Ye J, et al. Transcatheter valve-in-valve implantation for failed surgical bioprosthetic valves. J Am Coll Cardiol 2011;58: 2196–209.

50. Osten MD, Feindel C, Greutmann M, et al. Transcatheter aortic valve implantation for high risk patients with severe aortic stenosis using the Edwards Sapien balloon-expandable bioprosthesis: a single centre study with immediate and medium-term outcomes. Catheter Cardiovasc Interv 2010; 75:475–85.

51. Head SJ, Dewey TM, Mack MJ. Fungal endocarditis after transfemoral aortic valve implantation. Catheter Cardiovasc Interv 2011;78:1017–9.

52. Kidane AG, Burriesci G, Cornejo P, et al. Current developments and future prospects for heart valve replacement therapy. J Biomed Mater Res B Appl Biomater 2009;88:290–303.

53. Ghanbari H, Viatge H, Kidane AG, et al. Polymeric heart valves: new materials, emerging hopes. Trends Biotechnol 2009;27:359–67.

54. Wang Q, McGoron AJ, Bianco R, et al. In-vivo assessment of a novel polymer (SIBS) trileaflet heart valve. J Heart Valve Dis 2010;19:499–505.

55. Hyde JA, Chinn JA, Phillips RE Jr. Polymer heart valves. J Heart Valve Dis 1999;8:331–9.

56. Schoen FJ. Evolving concepts of cardiac valve dynamics: the continuum of development, functional

structure, pathobiology, and tissue engineering. Circulation 2008;118:1864–80.

57. Dohmen PM, Konertz W. Tissue-engineered heart valve scaffolds. Ann Thorac Cardiovasc Surg 2009;15:362–7.

58. Schoen FJ. Heart valve tissue engineering: quo vadis? Curr Opin Biotechnol 2011;22:698–705.

59. Dohmen PM, Lembcke A, Holinski S, et al. Ten years of clinical results with a tissue-engineered pulmonary valve. Ann Thorac Surg 2011;92:1308–14.

CARDIAC TRANSPLANT BIOPSIES

Gayle L. Winters, MD

KEYWORDS

- Endomyocardial biopsy • Transplant • Rejection • Peritransplant ischemic injury • Quilty effect
- Allograft coronary disease

ABSTRACT

The endomyocardial biopsy remains the gold standard for assessing the status of the transplanted heart. It is the most consistently reliable method for the diagnosis and grading of acute cellular and antibody-mediated rejection. Recognition of specimen artifacts and other biopsy findings such as ischemic injury, Quilty effect, infection, and post-transplant lymphoproliferative disorder is important for accurate biopsy interpretation and differentiation from rejection. The endomyocardial biopsy provides important diagnostic information essential for optimal management of cardiac transplant recipients.

Key Points
BIOPSY REQUIREMENTS FOR EVALUATION OF CARDIAC TRANSPLANT BIOPSIES

- Four (minimum 3) samples of myocardium
- Each sample consists of at least 50% myocardium (not fat, thrombus or fibrous tissue)
- Large samples should *not* be divided to achieve the required pieces
- Three slides/three sections per slide stained with H & E
- No additional special stains routinely required

OVERVIEW OF CARDIAC TRANSPLANT BIOPSIES

The endomyocardial biopsy has been the main method of assessing the status of the heart allograft for over four decades.

- The sensitivity of the endomyocardial biopsy is high (85 to 100%)
- The complication rate of endomyocardial biopsy is low (1 to 2%).[1–3]

Although the diagnosis of rejection is obviously foremost, additional biopsy findings such as ischemic injury, infection, post-transplant lymphoproliferative disorder (PTLD), disease recurrence, and changes secondary to allograft coronary disease can provide useful information for clinicians. Over the years, numerous non-invasive methods, and more recently, blood-based genetic profiling methods, have been proposed to replace some or all biopsies.[4–6] However, to date, the endomyocardial biopsy remains the gold standard for the diagnosis and grading of acute rejection and the assessment of other biopsy findings important in guiding the clinical management of heart transplant recipients.[7]

SPECIMEN ADEQUACY AND PROCESSING

- The first step in assessment of the post-transplant endomyocardial biopsy is to ensure that an adequate specimen has been received and that it is processed appropriately.
- Biopsies are typically obtained percutaneously from the right ventricle using a catheter-type instrument called a bioptome under fluoroscopic or echocardiographic guidance.
- Ideally, four (minimum of three) separate tissue samples should be obtained for light microscopy (**Fig. 1**) and each sample should consist

Department of Pathology, Brigham and Women's Hospital, Harvard Medical School, 75 Francis Street, Boston, MA 02115, USA
E-mail address: gwinters@partners.org

Surgical Pathology 5 (2012) 371–400
doi:10.1016/j.path.2012.04.003
1875-9181/12/$ – see front matter © 2012 Elsevier Inc. All rights reserved.

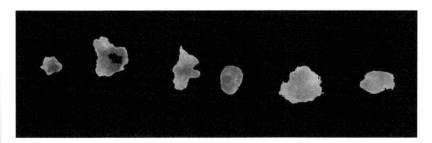

Fig. 1. Endomyocardial biopsy, gross. This is an adequate biopsy specimen consisting of 6 pieces of endomyocardial tissue ranging in size from 0.2 to 0.4 cm.

of at least 50% myocardium and not fat, thrombus, or fibrous tissue.[8]

- Large samples should not be cut to obtain the required number of samples since this practice defeats the purpose of obtaining representative samples of different areas of the myocardium.
- Samples are routinely placed in 10% neutral buffered formalin for paraffin embedding and processing.
- All samples may be wrapped or placed in a tissue bag and embedded together in the same cassette.
- Three slides with three sections per slides are stained with Hematoxylin and Eosin (H & E) (**Fig. 2**). No additional special stains are routinely required.

Assessment of antibody-mediated rejection may be done by either immunoperoxidase or immunofluorescence methods.[9] Immunoperoxidase staining for C4d and, in some institutions CD68, are performed on sections cut from the paraffin block. This method allows for staining localization and distribution of all pieces examined by H & E staining. If immunofluorescence is to be performed for C4d and/or C3d, an additional piece of myocardium should be obtained and either frozen or placed in an appropriate solution (Zeus or Michel's) since formalin fixation introduces confounding levels of autofluorescence.

BIOPSY PROTOCOLS

Transplant recipients undergo regularly scheduled biopsies according to specific protocols set by each transplant center. In general, biopsies are performed more frequently (ie, weekly) during the early post-transplant period. The interval between biopsies increases with time after transplantation reaching a frequency of one or two times annually after 1 year. Some transplant centers discontinue routine surveillance biopsies after a set period of time ranging from 6 months to 5 years.[10–14] The frequency of biopsies, however, may be increased if there is a change in the clinical status of the recipient or if acute rejection has been detected on a previous biopsy.

The protocol for assessing antibody-mediated rejection varies greatly between institutions.[15] Some institutions assess every biopsy, some assess all biopsies during the early post-transplant period, and some assess biopsies only when indicated by histologic findings and/or clinical scenarios. The latest ISHLT Consensus Conference recommends staining two biopsies in the first post-transplant month and then according to the center's circulating donor-specific antibody evaluation schedule. Immunostaining for C4d should be avoided during the first 2 post-transplant weeks because perioperative issues, especially ischemic injury, may confound staining and interpretation.[16]

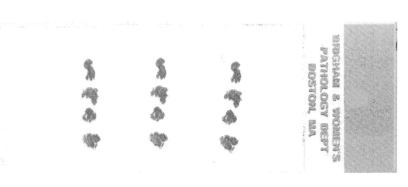

Fig. 2. Endomyocardial biopsy, histologic slide. Paraffin-embedded biopsy pieces have been sectioned with 3 levels per slide and stained with Hematoxylin and Eosin.

ACUTE CELLULAR REJECTION

MORPHOLOGY

Acute cellular rejection (**Fig. 3**) is characterized by an inflammatory cell infiltrate, which may be associated with damage to the myocardium and/or the vasculature.[17,18] The inflammatory infiltrate is predominantly lymphocytic (a mixture of CD4 and CD8 T cells) but may include macrophages and occasional eosinophils. In the most severe forms of rejection, the infiltrate is polymorphous, including neutrophils, eosinophils, and lymphocytes. Plasma cells are extremely rare in acute rejection and an abundance of plasma cells suggests an alternative process such as ischemic injury.

Myocardial damage or injury, originally called "myocyte necrosis," may be difficult to identify but is an important feature in grading rejection. Indeed, immune-mediated damage is generally an apoptosis-driven process that may be difficult to visualize by standard histology. In mild forms of rejection, "damage" is often represented histologically by encroachment of inflammatory cells along the perimeter of myocytes, partial "replacement" of myocytes by aggregates of inflammatory cells, or architectural distortion. In severe forms of rejection, myocyte damage and even distinguishable cell necrosis (likely secondary to vascular damage) is more obvious. In addition, vascular injury to small vessels results in hemorrhage and edema.

GRADING FOR ACUTE CELLULAR REJECTION

International Society for Heart and Lung Transplantation

Because the clinical therapeutic response to rejection should be proportional to the intensity of biopsy

Key Features
ACUTE CELLULAR REJECTION

- Mononuclear (lymphocytic) infiltrate ± myocyte damage

- ISHLT grading is based on the "worst" area of the biopsy

- "Multifocal" describes discrete areas of cellular infiltrate with or without myocyte damage with intervening uninvolved myocardium

- "Diffuse" pattern involves nearly the entire tissue fragment and the majority of tissue fragments are usually involved

pathology, the pathologist uses a grading system to consistently communicate biopsy findings to the transplant clinician. An international grading system for cardiac allograft biopsies was adopted by the International Society for Heart and Lung Transplantation (ISHLT) in 1990 to facilitate communication between clinicians and investigators, to enable comparison of treatment regimens and outcomes, to facilitate multicenter clinical trials, and to promote further studies to determine the clinical significance of various histologic patterns.[19] The grading system was widely adopted and served the transplant community well for over a decade. A multidisciplinary review of the grading system was undertaken under the direction of the ISHLT in 2004 to address challenges and inconsistencies in its use, to consider changes in rejection incidence and treatment practices, and to incorporate advances in medical knowledge.[8,20–32]

The outcome of the consensus conference was revision of the 1990 working formulation for

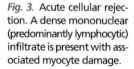

Fig. 3. Acute cellular rejection. A dense mononuclear (predominantly lymphocytic) infiltrate is present with associated myocyte damage.

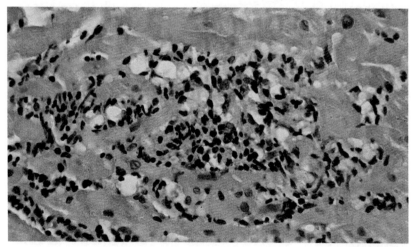

Table 1
ISHLT standardized cardiac biopsy grading
Grading of acute cellular rejection

2004		1990	
Grade 0R	**No Rejection**	**Grade 0**	**No Rejection**
Grade 1R Mild	Interstitial and/or perivascular infiltrate with up to 1 focus of myocyte damage	Grade 1 Mild A – Focal	Focal perivascular and/or interstitial infiltrate without myocyte damage
		B – Diffuse	Diffuse infiltrate without myocyte damage
		Grade 2 Moderate (focal)	One focus of infiltrate with associated myocyte damage
Grade 2R Moderate	Two or more foci of infiltrate with associated myocyte damage	Grade 3 Moderate A – Focal	Multifocal infiltrate with myocyte damage
Grade 3R Severe	Diffuse infiltrate with multifocal myocyte damage ± edema, ± hemorrhage ± vasculitis	B – Diffuse	Diffuse infiltrate with myocyte damage
		Grade 4 Severe	Diffuse polymorphous infiltrate with extensive myocyte damage ± edema, ± hemorrhage + vasculitis

cellular rejection and includes an "R" after the rejection grade indicating the 2004 revision. The major changes from 1990 to 2004 were that:

- 7 grades were reduced to 4 grades

- 1990 Grade 2 rejection was combined with 1990 Grades 1A and 1B into a single grade for mild rejection, Grade 1R.

Although the ISHLT 2004 grading system is officially endorsed by the ISHLT, a survey of pathology

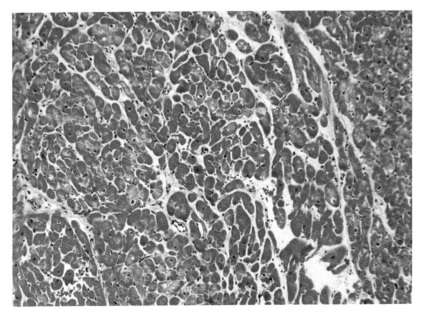

Fig. 4. ISHLT Grade 0R. This is a biopsy without evidence of rejection. Occasional nuclei present within the interstitium represent nuclei of endothelial cells, fibroblasts, and a rare lymphocyte.

Fig. 5. ISHLT Grade 1R. This is a biopsy with mild rejection. A perivascular lymphocytic infiltrate without myocyte damage is present in (*A*) (1990 ISHLT Grade 1A). An interstitial lymphocytic infiltrate without myocyte damage is present in (*B*) (1990 ISHLT Grade 1B). A single focus of lymphocytic infiltrate with associated myocyte damage (*arrows*) is present in (*C*) (1990 ISHLT Grade 2).

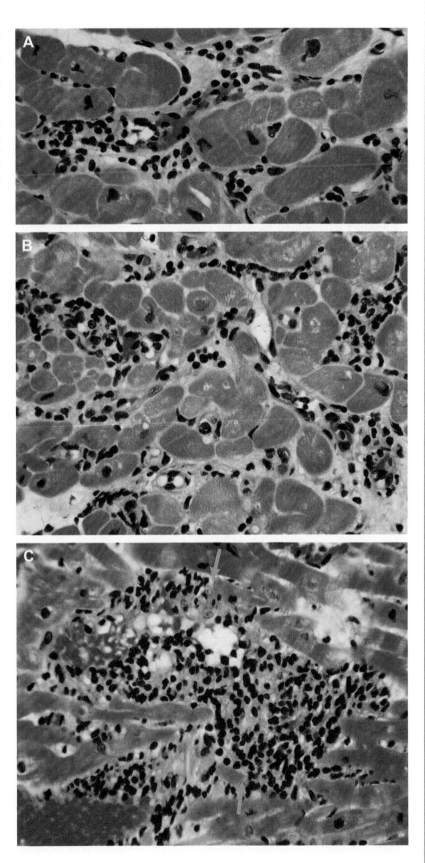

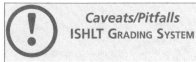

Caveats/Pitfalls
ISHLT GRADING SYSTEM

! Designed for endomyocardial biopsies and not autopsy or explanted hearts

! Based on histologic findings before any treatment except for maintenance immuno-suppression

! Does not recognize "resolving" or "resolved" rejection; any residual rejection and/or healing should be given a rejection grade

! Provides standardized format for conveying biopsy findings but does not attempt to incorporate clinical parameters or recommend treatment

practice in North America indicates that only 45% of heart transplant centers use ISHLT 2004 exclusively, 40% use ISHLT 2004 in conjunction with ISHLT 1990, and 12% retain the use of ISHLT 1990 exclusively.[33] Therefore, both grading systems

are presented in Table 1, however, discussion in the text refers to the ISHLT 2004 Grading System. The ISHLT grading system is intended for application to biopsy specimens, and is not intended to assess autopsy or explanted hearts.

Grades in ISHLT 2004 Grading System

Grade 0R
This grade represents no evidence of rejection. Normal myocardium contains a small number of lymphocytes and other interstitial cells which may resemble lymphocytes in cross section. These findings should not be interpreted as rejection. Lymphocytes within blood vessels, fat, and adipose tissue also do not constitute rejection (Fig. 4).

Grade 1R
This grade represents mild rejection. Perivascular and/or interstitial lymphocytes may be present in one or more foci in one or more biopsy fragments. Associated myocyte damage may be present in up to one focus (Fig. 5).

Grade 2R
This grade represents moderate rejection. Multiple (2 or more) foci of lymphocytic infiltrates

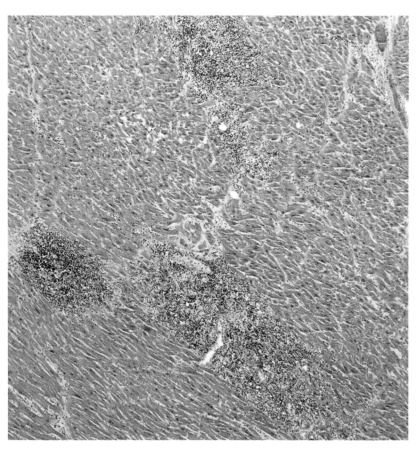

Fig. 6. ISHLT Grade 2R (1990 ISHLT Grade 3A). This is a biopsy with moderate rejection. Multiple foci ($\geq$2) of lymphocytic infiltrates with associated myocyte damage are present. These foci are separated by uninvolved areas of myocardium.

Fig. 7. ISHLT Grade 3R. This is a biopsy with severe rejection. In (*A*) (1990 ISHLT Grade 3B), there is a diffuse lymphocytic infiltrate with associated myocyte damage involving most biopsy pieces. In (*B*) (1990 ISHLT Grade 4), there is extensive infiltration along with edema and myocyte damage. Higher power, (*C*) reveals a polymorphous infiltrate with edema and extensive myocyte damage.

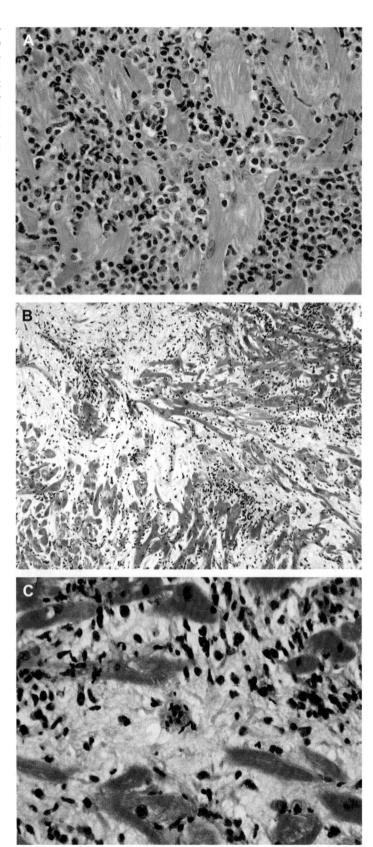

associated with myocyte damage are present. These foci may be distributed in one or more than one of the biopsy pieces. Intervening foci of uninvolved myocardium can be identified (Fig. 6).

Grade 3R

This grade represents severe rejection. A diffuse polymorphous inflammatory infiltrate with widespread myocyte damage is present in all, or nearly all, biopsy pieces and may involve the endocardium. Edema and hemorrhage are usually present and vasculitis is frequently seen (Fig. 7).

INDICATIONS FOR THERAPEUTIC INTERVENTION FOR CELLULAR REJECTION

In most transplant centers, the threshold for augmenting immunosuppression is Grade 2R rejection. Grade 3R rejection is universally treated aggressively (eg, with intravenous steroids or anti-CD3 monoclonal antibodies) and is often the most difficult to reverse. Grade 1R rejection may elicit no treatment response, or clinicians may opt to rebiopsy the patient earlier than scheduled by protocol and/or optimize immunosuppression therapy by checking blood levels and hemodynamics.

ANTIBODY-MEDIATED REJECTION

Antibody-mediated rejection (AMR) is an evolving and controversial issue in cardiac transplantation.[34–37] AMR was originally recognized as a clinicopathologic entity characterized by

1. Cardiac dysfunction in the absence of cellular rejection or ischemic injury
2. Characteristic histologic features on endomyocardial biopsy (see below)
3. Positive immunoperoxidase staining for the complement component C4d
4. Presence of circulating anti-donor antibodies.

It often occurs in sensitized patients (including those with previous transplantation, transfusion or pregnancy, and previous ventricular assist device use) and is associated with worse graft survival.[37,38] The incidence of AMR is highly variable between transplant centers, but most agree that the incidence in heart transplant recipients is low (<5%).

MORPHOLOGY AND IMMUNOSTAINING

Histologic features described in AMR include interstitial edema, endothelial cell swelling, and intravascular macrophages (Fig. 8). These findings,

however, do not always correlate with C4d positivity[39] and for this reason, use of these histologic findings in screening biopsies for AMR has been questioned.[40,41]

The choice of which antibodies to use in assessing AMR depends on whether immunohistochemistry (IC) (on paraffin embedded tissue) or immunofluorescence (IF) (on frozen tissue) is used. C4d is the most commonly used antibody for IC (Fig. 9A) with C3d and CD68 (macrophage marker) used by some centers.[15] Antibodies recommended for IF are C4d (see Fig. 9B) and C3d with HLA staining used for identification of capillary structures and evaluation of vascular damage as needed. Many transplant centers have developed their own preferences for panels of antibodies which may include: CD31, CD34, CD3, C4d, C3d, CD68, immunoglobulins, and fibrin. In the interpretation of antibody staining, *only* the interstitial capillaries should be assessed (not venules, arterioles, small arteries, Quilty lesions, myocardial scars, or myocardium). Staining should be moderate or intense and multifocal or diffuse to be considered positive. Thus, faint, focal staining is not considered positive.[16]

GRADING FOR ANTIBODY-MEDIATED REJECTION

The ISHLT 2004 Grading System recommends reporting whether AMR is absent (AMR 0) or present (AMR 1).[8] A more recent AMR Consensus Conference sponsored by the ISHLT recommends separating "pathologic AMR" from the clinical components and proposed the following categories to permit the accumulation of additional data and experience (Table 2).[16]

pAMR 0: Negative for pathologic AMR. Both the histologic findings and immunopathologic studies are negative.

pAMR 1 (H+): Histologic findings are consistent with AMR, however immunopathologic studies are negative.

pAMR 1 (I+): Histologic findings are negative, however immunopathologic studies are positive for AMR.

pAMR 2: Pathologic AMR. Both histologic and immunopathologic findings are positive for AMR.

pAMR 3: Severe Pathologic AMR. This category includes rare cases of severe AMR with marked edema, interstitial hemorrhage, capillary fragmentation, and endothelial cell pyknosis and/or karyorrhexis in addition to a mixed inflammatory infiltrate. These cases are associated with severe hemodynamic dysfunction and poor clinical outcomes.

Fig. 8. Antibody-mediated rejection. On low power, (*A*) there is a "busy" appearance to the interstitium that contains a polymorphous infiltrate without significant myocyte damage. Higher power, (*B*) reveals endothelial cell swelling, perivascular edema, and occasional intravascular macrophages.

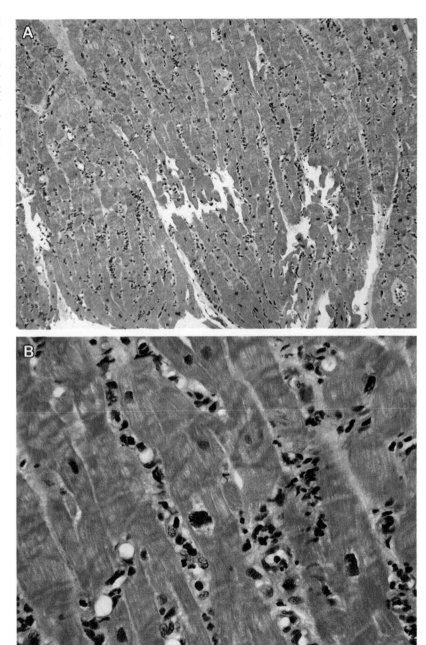

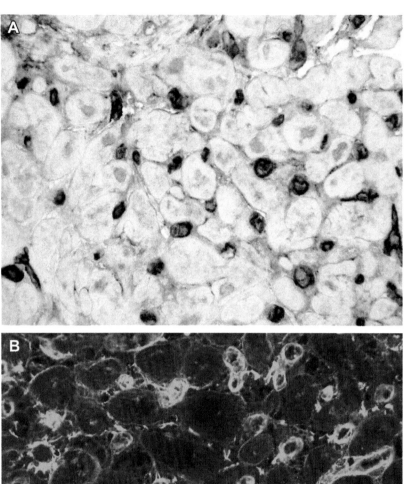

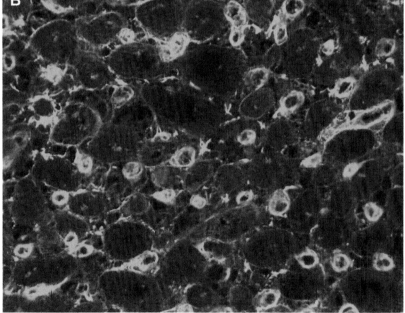

Fig. 9. Antibody-mediated rejection. Immunoperoxidase staining, (*A*) and immunofluorescence staining, (*B*) for C4d reveals strong, diffuse positivity of the interstitial capillaries.

Table 2
ISHLT recommendations for acute antibody-mediated rejection

	2011		2004
pAMR 0	Negative for pathologic AMR. Both histologic findings and immunopathologic studies are negative	AMR 0	Negative for acute antibody-mediated rejection. No histologic or immunopathologic features of AMR
pAMR 1 (H+)	Histologic findings are consistent with AMR, however immunopathologic studies are negative	AMR 1	Positive for AMR. Histologic features of AMR. Positive immunofluorescence or immunoperoxidase staining for AMR (positive C4d, CD68)
pAMR 1 (I+)	Histologic findings are negative; however immunopathologic studies are positive for AMR		
pAMR 2	Pathologic AMR. Both histologic and immunopathologic findings are positive for AMR		
pAMR 3	Severe pathologic AMR. Includes rare cases with marked edema, interstitial hemorrhage, capillary fragmentation, and endothelial cell pyknosis and/or karyorrhexis in addition to a mixed inflammatory infiltrate. Associated with severe dysfunction and poor outcome		

INDICATIONS FOR THERAPEUTIC INTERVENTION FOR ANTIBODY-MEDIATED REJECTION

Treatment of AMR is also controversial.[42] Most transplant centers treat AMR (positive C4d staining on endomyocardial biopsy and positive serum antibodies in a hemodynamically compromised patient) with plasmapheresis. Less clear is the appropriate clinical response for a patient who is clinically doing well yet has positive C4d staining on endomyocardial biopsy with or without characteristic histology and/or positive donor specific antibodies. Whether this represents "subclinical" AMR which may impact allograft/patient longevity and/or contribute to allograft vasculopathy remains unknown.

OTHER POST-TRANSPLANT BIOPSY FINDINGS

PRIMARY DISEASE RECURRENCE IN THE ALLOGRAFT

Diseases known to recur in the heart allograft include amyloidosis, sarcoidosis, Chagas Disease, giant cell myocarditis, and hemochromatosis.[43–45] Patients with sarcoidosis and amyloidosis have undergone successful transplantation, although recurrence of the disease in the transplanted heart, or progression of the disease systemically may limit the long-term benefits.[46] A case of non-HFE hemochromatosis first diagnosed in the explanted heart recurred within 6 months of transplantation.[47] Although patients with active lymphocytic myocarditis at the time of transplant were thought to have increased frequency and severity of acute rejection, more recent outcome of patients transplanted for myocarditis was found to be similar to that of patients with other forms of dilated cardiomyopathy.[48] Whether the pathology in the transplanted heart represents rejection or recurrent myocarditis cannot be readily distinguished since the histologic appearances and pathologic mechanisms are identical.

PERITRANSPLANT ISCHEMIC INJURY

Early Post-Transplant Ischemic Injury

Ischemic injury is a frequent finding on endomyocardial biopsies obtained during the early post-transplant period and may be diagnosed by conventional histologic criteria.[49,50] The morphologic characteristics of early ischemic injury include coagulative myocyte necrosis, fat necrosis, and a mixed cellular infiltrate (Fig. 10). The earliest finding (1 to 2 weeks) of coagulative myocyte necrosis often extends to the endocardial surface, unlike a typical myocardial infarction which contains an intervening zone of viable myocardium perfused directly by blood in the ventricular cavity.

Healing Phase of Post-Transplant Ischemic Injury

Subsequent biopsies (2 to 4 weeks or more) may reveal the healing phase of this early ischemic injury (Fig. 11). It is characterized by a mixed inflammatory infiltrate consisting of neutrophils, macrophages, lymphocytes and plasma cells. At this point, confusion with acute rejection may occur (Fig. 12).

The healing inflammatory response following ischemic injury is predominantly in the interstitium or perivascular spaces, not encroaching on, and usually with a clear separation from, adjacent myocytes. Cellular debris is frequently present in the inflammatory foci. Healing fat necrosis and myocyte vacuolization in the adjacent myocardium are often present. The healing response to early ischemic injury may be protracted due to the anti-inflammatory effects of immunosuppression and has been observed up to 6 months after transplantation in some patients.

BIOPSY SITE

Obtaining tissue from a previous biopsy site is the most common sampling artifact in biopsy interpretation. The average transplant patient undergoes

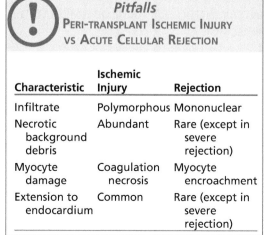

Fig. 10. Peri-transplant ischemic injury, early. Within the first 2 to 3 weeks after transplantation, coagulative myocyte necrosis, (*A*) and fat necrosis, (*B*) are common biopsy findings.

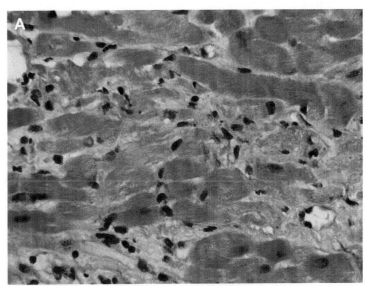

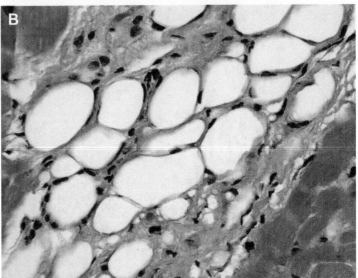

Fig. 11. Peri-transplant ischemic injury, healing. As peri-transplant ischemic injury heals, a polymorphous inflammatory infiltrate is present. There has been extensive ischemic damage to the myocytes with necrotic debris in the background.

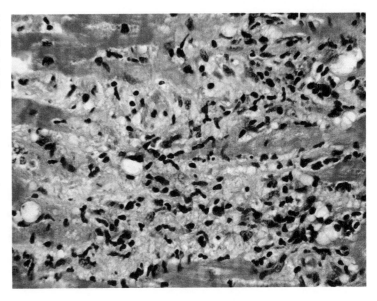

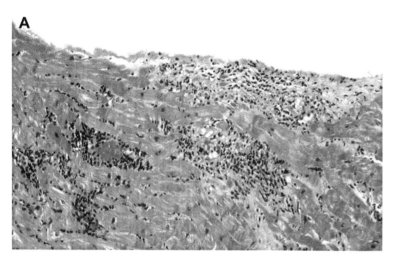

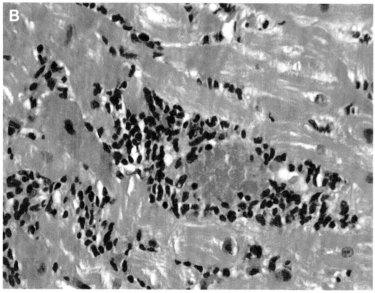

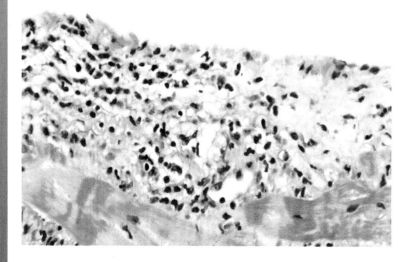

Fig. 12. Comparison of peritransplant ischemic injury and acute rejection. On low power, (A) acute rejection (dense infiltrate) is present on the left; healing ischemic injury (polymorphous infiltrate) is present on the right. Healing ischemic injury, which occurs during transport when there is no blood in the ventricular cavity, often extends to the endocardium. High power of acute rejection, (B) and healing ischemic injury, (C).

up to 20 biopsies during the first year after transplantation. Due to the rigid structure of the bioptome and relatively constant configuration of the right ventricle, the bioptome tends to follow a similar path with each succeeding biopsy in any given patient. The histology of the biopsy site reflects the degree of healing that has occurred. Immediately following a biopsy procedure, fresh thrombus may overlie areas of acute myocyte injury and hemorrhage (**Fig. 13**A). Progressive healing results in granulation tissue or fibrosis, often containing a leukocytic infiltrate and thick-walled vessels with myocyte disarray at the periphery (see **Fig. 13**B). The mixed nature of the healing inflammatory infiltrate and the

myocyte disarray frequently present at the periphery of the biopsy site aid in rendering a correct interpretation of the findings.

QUILTY EFFECT

Endocardial infiltrates, termed Quilty effect after the first patient in whom they were observed, are raised cellular aggregates arising from the endocardium.[51–55] They are easily accessible to the bioptome and are present in 10 to 20% of post-transplant biopsies. These lesions can appear at any time during the post-transplant course and, once present, tend to persist in any given patient. The etiology of Quilty effect and relationship to

Fig. 13. Biopsy site. Re-biopsy of a previous biopsy site is common. In (*A*) the biopsy site is recent, consisting of organizing thrombus. In (*B*) the biopsy site is remote characterized by fibrosis with neovascularization and myocyte disarray at the base.

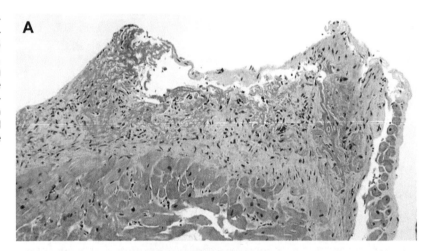

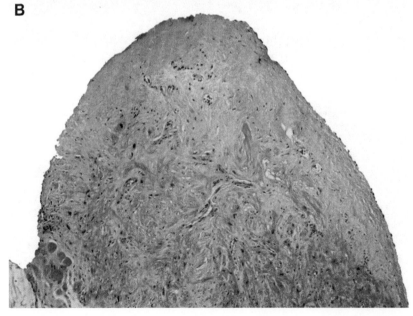

acute rejection, if any, are unknown. However, the lesion is traditionally considered distinct from rejection, and does not require any change in the immunosuppression regimen. It also does not appear to be related to viral infection or post-transplant lymphoproliferative disorders. Quilty effect consists of densely cellular endocardial nodules composed of lymphocytes (including B cells), admixed with macrophages, plasma cells and numerous small blood vessels. The infiltrates may be confined to the endocardium (Fig. 14A), or may extend into the underlying myocardium where associated myocyte damage can be present (see Fig. 14B). Even with associated myocyte damage, Quilty lesions do not mandate adjustment of immunosuppression.

INFECTION IN HEART TRANSPLANTS

Immunosuppressed cardiac transplant recipients are at increased risk of opportunistic infection that can also involve the allograft.[56] Organisms encountered on endomyocardial biopsy specimens include cytomegalovirus (CMV) (Fig. 15), Toxoplasma gondii (Fig. 16), and Chagas disease (Fig. 17). These infections can occur as either primary or reactivated infection. The accompanying

A

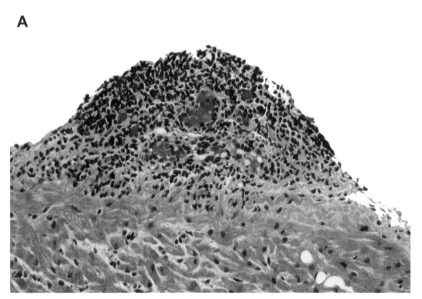

B

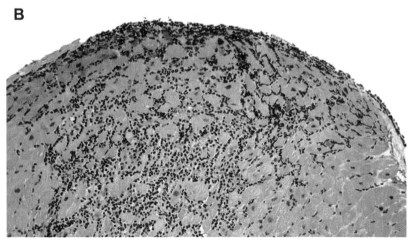

Fig. 14. Quilty effect. Quilty effect is an endocardially-based lymphocytic infiltrate, often with prominent vascularity. It may be confined to the endocardium, (A) or extend into the underlying myocardium, (B) where it may be associated with myocyte damage.

Fig. 15. Cytomegalovirus (CMV). CMV inclusions (*arrows*) are present within myocytes.

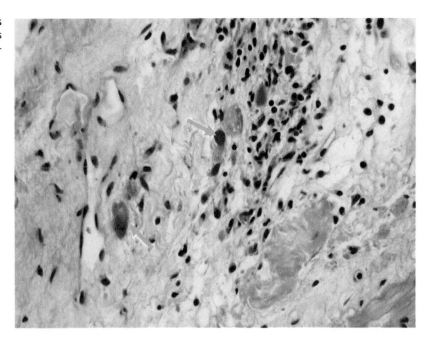

cellular infiltrate is highly variable and in some cases infection may incite little or no inflammatory reaction. In suspected cases, immunohistochemistry to detect viral antigens, in situ hybridization, and/or polymerase chain reaction to detect DNA may be useful adjuncts to histopathology. Toxoplasmosis can also be stained by periodic acid-Schiff (PAS) staining and immunoperoxidase techniques.

Fig. 16. Toxoplasmosis. Toxoplasma cysts are present within a myocyte.

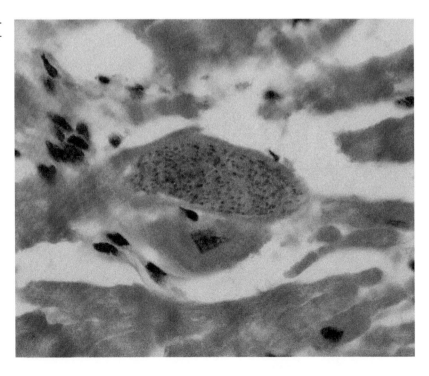

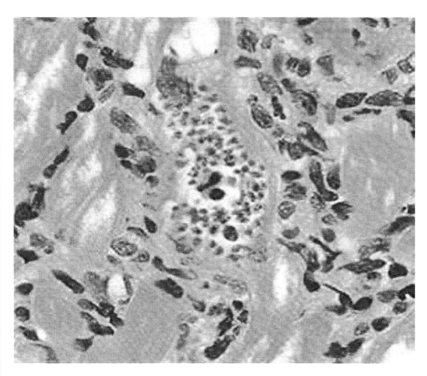

Fig. 17. Chagas disease. Trypanosoma cruzi organisms are present within a myocyte.

Infection in patients surviving at least 1 year after transplantation is less common; there is often a precipitating event (ie, rejection) requiring augmentation of immunosuppression that precedes the development of infection. As in any immunosuppressed patient, fungal infections may occur and, when disseminated, may include the heart allograft (**Fig. 18**).

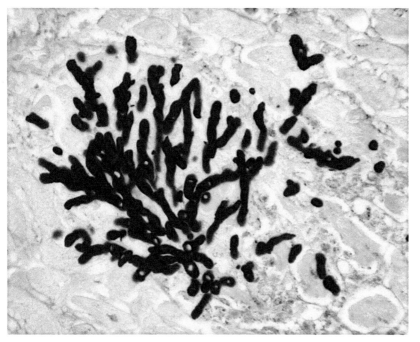

Fig. 18. Fungus (Aspergillus). Disseminated fungal infections in an immunocompromised host may involve the myocardium (Silver stain).

POST-TRANSPLANT LYMPHOPROLIFERATIVE DISORDER

Post-transplant lymphoproliferative disorder (PTLD) is often an aggressive neoplasm which occurs in approximately 2% of heart transplant recipients and is likely related to the intensity of immunosuppressive regimen.[57] It can involve the allograft[58] where it must be differentiated from acute rejection, but more frequently it involves extranodal sites such as the lung, gastrointestinal tract, central nervous system and soft tissues. The lymphocytes are large and atypical with prominent and often multiple nuclei, mitoses, and individual cell necrosis (Fig. 19). Most PTLDs are disorders of B-cell origin (vs T-cells in rejection), ranging from benign polyclonal B-cell hyperplasias to malignant monoclonal lymphomas with clonal chromosomal abnormalities. EBV has been strongly associated with PTLDs. Immunosuppressive drugs used to prevent allograft rejection suppress the T-cell responses that would normally suppress EBV-induced B-cell proliferations. Treatment involves reducing the immunosuppression intensity and can also include traditional chemotherapy. Mortality rates as high as 60 to 100% have been cited. Characteristics associated with poorer survival include diagnosis within the first year posttransplant and monoclonal tumors.

ALLOGRAFT CORONARY DISEASE AND LATE ISCHEMIC INJURY

Allograft coronary disease is a diffuse proliferative process that results in obstruction of the epicardial and/or intramyocardial arteries with secondary ischemic injury to the myocardium.[59–62] It is characterized by an immune-mediated concentric intimal proliferation composed largely of smooth muscle cells (Fig. 20). By endomyocardial biopsy, it is unusual to obtain vessels large enough to assess this process, however the secondary changes to the myocardium are more readily apparent (see below).

SUBENDOCARDIAL MYOCYTE VACUOLIZATION

Subendocardial myocyte vacuolization (SEMV)[63] (Fig. 21) is a potentially reversible change resulting from chronic ischemia. In the immediate post-transplant period and extending for 2 to 3 months, SEMV more commonly reflects perioperative ischemia. However, the finding of SEMV one year or more post-transplant should raise the possibility of allograft coronary disease and may provide an early clue to the existence of this disease.

MICROINFARCTS

Acute, healing, or healed subendocardial microinfarcts (Fig. 22) may be detected on endomyocardial biopsy and suggest small vessel involvement by allograft coronary disease.

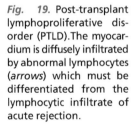

Fig. 19. Post-transplant lymphoproliferative disorder (PTLD).The myocardium is diffusely infiltrated by abnormal lymphocytes (*arrows*) which must be differentiated from the lymphocytic infiltrate of acute rejection.

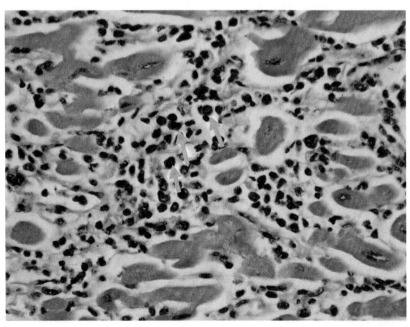

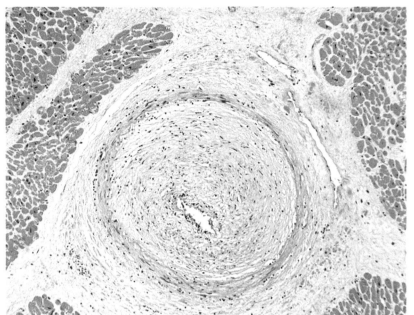

Fig. 20. Allograft coronary disease, artery. A small intra-myocardial artery contains diffuse fibrous intimal proliferation.

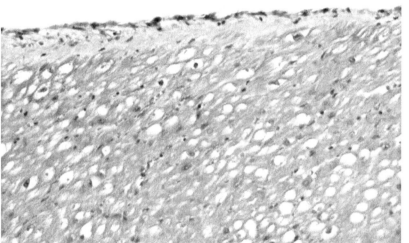

Fig. 21. Allograft coronary disease, subendocardial myocyte vacuolization (SEMV). First described at the periphery of myocardial infarctions, SEMV is characteristic of reversible ischemic injury.

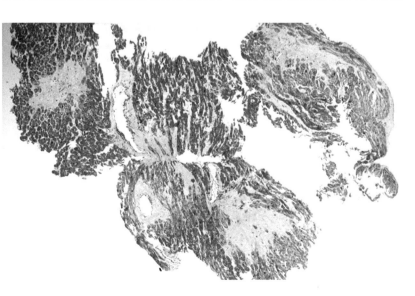

Fig. 22. Allograft coronary disease, microinfarcts. Occlusion of small arteries by allograft coronary disease may result in microinfarct(s) in various stages of healing. In this biopsy, multiple healed microinfarcts are present.

TISSUE ARTIFACTS

EDEMA

Handling and processing of the biopsy specimen may result in artificial separation of myocytes by empty white spaces. In true edema, proteinaceous material is often detected between myocytes. Although true edema is a component of some pathologic conditions such as severe acute rejection, care should be taken is diagnosing edema in the absence of other histologic findings. True edema may be associated with inadequate calcineurin-inhibitor (eg, cyclosporine) levels, with secondary elevations in interleukin-2 that can increase vascular permeability (Fig. 23).

Differential Diagnosis
TISSUE ARTIFACTS

- Edema
- Hemorrhage
- Thrombus
- Contraction Bands
- Telescoping
- Intravascular Lymphocytes
- Fat/Mesothelial Cells
- Foreign Body
- Tissue Other Than Myocardium

Fig. 23. Edema. True interstitial edema often has eosinophilic material in the spaces between myocytes and must be distinguished from artifactual separation of myocytes resulting from processing.

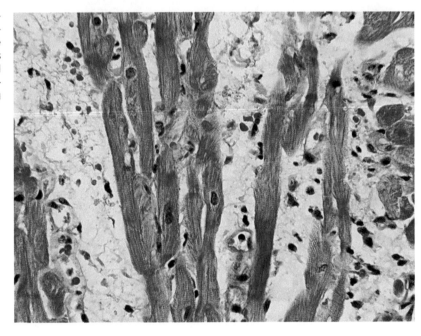

HEMORRHAGE

Hemorrhage may occur secondary to the trauma of the biopsy process. Similar to edema, hemorrhage may be part of pathologic processes but should not be considered diagnostically important in the absence of other histologic findings (Fig. 24).

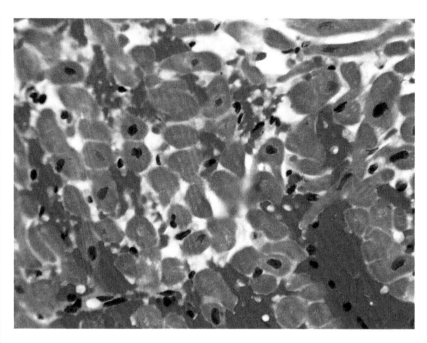

Fig. 24. Hemorrhage. Hemorrhage may result from the biopsy procedure and must be distinguished from hemorrhage which occurs as part of severe rejection. In the latter, additional histologic findings such as edema, inflammatory infiltrates, and myocyte damage are typically present.

THROMBUS

Although mural thrombus may be part of pathologic conditions, thrombus on endomyocardial biopsy is often associated with a previous biopsy site. It should be distinguished from necrotic myocardium which it sometimes can resemble and should not be counted as a piece of myocardium for the purpose of specimen adequacy (Fig. 25).

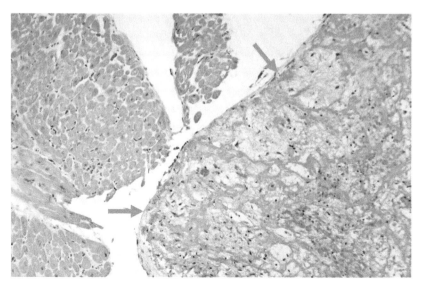

Fig. 25. Thrombus. Particularly in patients who have undergone previous biopsies, thrombus (*arrows*) from a previous biopsy site may be obtained on subsequent biopsies and does not necessarily imply luminal thrombus. It also must be differentiated from necrotic myocardium.

CONTRACTION BANDS

Contraction bands may occur as a result of the biopsy procedure and placement of viable tissue specimens in a cold solution where they undergo a final tetanic contraction. These contraction bands often span several myocytes and do not indicate myocardial ischemic injury (**Fig. 26**).[64]

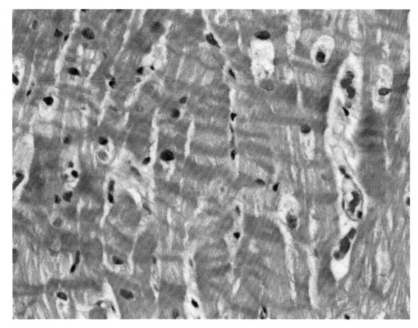

Fig. 26. Contraction bands. Contraction bands, particularly those spanning several myocytes are an artifact of biopsying the beating heart and do not represent myocardial ischemia or necrosis.

TELESCOPING

Sectioning of vessels may result in retraction of distal media within the lumen of the vessel. This is not of pathologic significance and should not be confused with an organized thrombus (**Fig. 27**).

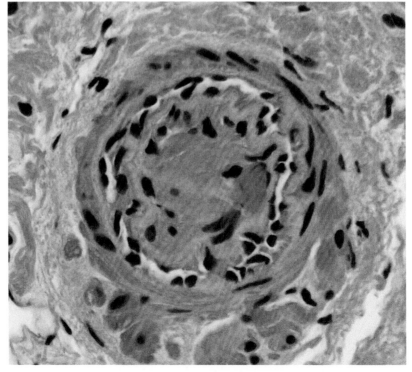

Fig. 27. Telescoping. Telescoping, or intussusception, of small vessels should not be mistaken for luminal thrombus or intimal thickening.

INTRAVASCULAR LYMPHOCYTES

Sectioning through tissue specimens may reveal collections of intravascular lymphocytes (usually intralymphatic) which should not be considered pathologic or to represent acute rejection (Fig. 28).

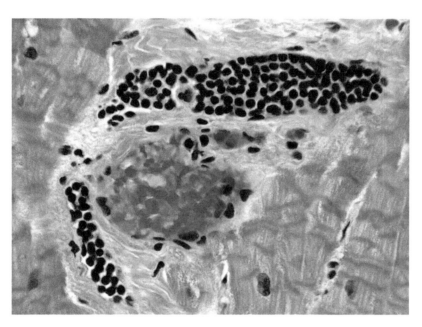

Fig. 28. Intravascular lymphocytes. Accumulations of intravascular (intralymphatic) lymphocytes should not be interpreted as acute rejection.

FAT/MESOTHELIAL CELLS

Intramyocardial adipose tissue is normally present within the right ventricle of many patients where it is within reach of the bioptome. Fat alone within endomyocardial biopsy tissue is of no diagnostic significance. The presence of mesothelial cells, however, is diagnostic of perforation and warrants notification of the clinicians caring for the patient (**Fig. 29**).

Fig. 29. Adipose tissue and mesothelial cells. Infiltration of the right ventricle by adipose tissue, (*A*) is common, may appear in endomyocardial biopsy specimens, and does not necessarily indicate myocardial perforation. The presence of mesothelial cells (*arrows*), however, (*B*) is diagnostic of myocardial perforation.

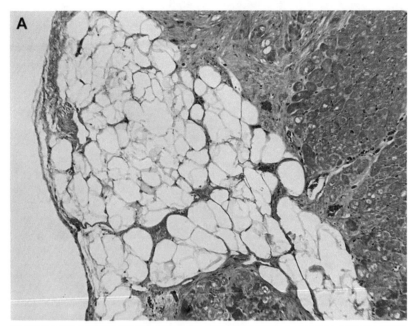

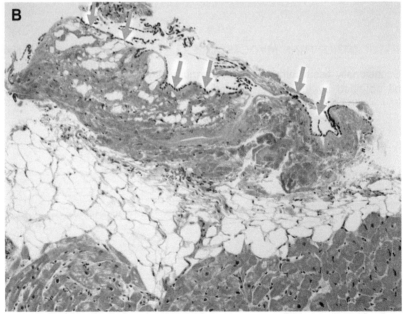

FOREIGN BODY

Foreign body giant cells in association with foreign material are sometimes present in endomyocardial biopsies from patients who have undergone previous biopsy procedures. This material is most likely cotton thread from gauze used to wipe the bioptome or fragments of catheter sheath (Fig. 30).

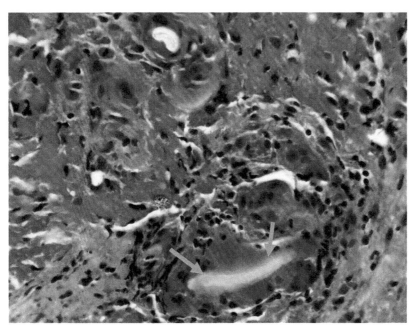

Fig. 30. Foreign body. Foreign material (*arrows*), often engulfed by foreign body giant cells may appear in endomyocardial biopsy specimens and frequently represents fragments of gauze used to wipe the bioptome in previous biopsy procedures.

TISSUE OTHER THAN MYOCARDIUM

Occasionally tissue other than myocardium may be obtained by the biopsy procedure. Valvular tissue, chordae tendineae, and liver have all been reported in biopsy specimens (Fig. 31).

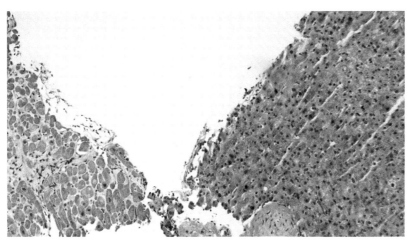

Fig. 31. Tissue other than myocardium. In rare instances, tissue other than myocardium may be biopsied. In this case, a fragment of liver is present on the right and myocardium is on the left. Fragments of tricuspid valve and chordae may also appear in endomyocardial biopsy specimens.

Fig. 32. Standardized sign-out form. Use of a standardized signout form provides consistency in reporting endomyocardial biopsy results, particularly when more than one pathologist interprets transplant biopsies. See discussion on following page.

TRANSPLANT ENDOMYOCARDIAL BIOPSY

CASE #BS_____-_____   RES _____   CARDIAC _____

E1 **RIGHT VENTRICULAR ENDOMYOCARDIAL BIOPSY**

(-) _____

Post-operative interval
E2 _____ days S/P cardiac transplantation.
E3 _____ weeks S/P cardiac transplantation.
E4 _____ months S/P cardiac transplantation.
E5 _____ years S/P cardiac transplantation.
E6 _____ years and _____ months S/P cardiac transplantation.

Cellular Rejection grading
E7 No evidence of rejection; ISHLT Grade 0 R.
E8 Interstitial and/or perivascular infiltrate with up to 1 focus of myocyte damage; ISHLT Grade 1 R, mild rejection.
E9 Two – three foci of lymphocytic infiltrates with myocyte damage; BWH Grade 1-2 R; (ISHLT Grade 2 R), mild to moderate rejection.
E10 Multiple foci (>3) of infiltrate with associated myocyte damage; ISHLT Grade 2 R, moderate rejection.
E11 Diffuse infiltrate with multifocal myocyte damage ± edema ± hemorrhage ± vasculitis; ISHLT Grade 3 R, severe rejection.
(-) _____

Antibody-Mediated Rejection (AMR)
E12 pAMR 0: Negative for pathologic AMR. Both histologic findings and immunopathologic studies are negative.
E13a pAMR 1 (H+): Histologic findings are consistent with AMR; however immunopathologic studies (C4d staining) are negative.
E13b pAMR 1 (I+): Histologic findings are negative for AMR; however immunopathologic studies (C4d staining) are positive for AMR.
E14 pAMR 2: Pathologic AMR. Both histological and immunopathologic (C4d) findings are positive for AMR.
E15 pAMR 3: Severe Pathologic AMR. AMR with marked edema, interstitial hemorrhage, capillary fragmentation, and endothelial cell pyknosis and/or karyorrhexis in addition to a mixed inflammatory infiltrate.

Other biopsy findings
E16 Tissue insufficient for definitive diagnosis.
E17   NOTE: No rejection is seen on _____ fragments of evaluable myocardium, however, the presence of less than three (3) fragments of evaluable myocardium is considered suboptimal to rule out rejection with a high degree of certainty.
E18   NOTE: _____ is seen on _____ fragments of evaluable myocardium, however the presence of less than three (3) fragments is considered suboptimal to rule out more severe rejection with a high degree of certainty.
E19 Focal coagulation necrosis.
E20 Multifocal coagulation necrosis.
E21 Confluent coagulation necrosis.
E22 Focal healing ischemic injury.
E23 Multifocal healing ischemic injury.
E24 Confluent healing ischemic injury.
E25 Focal healing injury.
E26 Multifocal healing injury.
E27 Focal fat necrosis.
E28 Old biopsy site.
E29 Foreign body giant cell reaction.
E30 Dystrophic calcification.
E31 No subendocardial myocyte vacuolization identified.
E32 Mild subendocardial myocyte vacuolization.
E33 Moderate subendocardial myocyte vacuolization.
E34 Severe subendocardial myocyte vacuolization.
E35 Quilty Effect
E36 Mesothelial cells present.
          NOTE: The presence of mesothelial cells on endomyocardial biopsy is diagnostic of cardiac perforation; clinical correlation is advised.
E37 See note.
(-) _____

Specimen adequacy
E38 _____ fragments of diagnostic myocardium.
E39 _____ fragments of fibrous tissue.
E40 _____ fragments of blood clot.
E41 _____ fragments of adipose tissue.
E42 _____ fragments too small to evaluate.
(-) _____

E43 _____, Cardiac Transplant Clinical Nurse Specialist, was notified of results on _____ at _____.
          (date)   (time)

COMMUNICATING TRANSPLANT BIOPSY RESULTS AND THE ROLE OF THE SURGICAL PATHOLOGIST

Transplant endomyocardial biopsy results should be communicated to the transplant clinician or their designee in a consistent manner. When more than one pathologist is responsible for interpreting and reporting biopsy results, use of a standardized form may provide consistency (**Fig. 32**). This form is easily computerized, saving transcription time and reducing typing errors. The use of standardized reports, however, should not prevent the pathologist from providing narrative description of difficult cases to the clinician and discussing such cases directly.

PROGNOSIS FOR CARDIAC TRANSPLANT RECIPIENTS

Cardiac transplantation represents the most definitive therapy for patients with end-stage heart failure. Between 1982 and 2009, over 97,000 heart transplants performed at over 300 heart transplant centers worldwide were recorded by the International Society for Heart and Lung Transplantation Transplant Registry.[65] In the last decade, between 3600 and 3850 heart transplants were registered each year and in 2011, the 100,000th heart transplant was performed. The number of patients bridged to transplant with mechanical circulatory support continues to increase, exceeding 30% of patients transplanted for the first time in 2009. Actuarial survival for cardiac transplant recipients is approximately 85% at one year, 70% at 5 years, and 50% at 10 years.

The clinical management of heart transplant recipients is guided, in part, by the pathologist who interprets the post-transplant endomyocardial biopsies. The diagnosis and grading of rejection allows for tailoring of immunosuppressive therapy. Equally important is the differentiation of other post-transplant biopsy findings from acute rejection so that transplant recipients are not over-immunosuppressed. Close collaboration between the pathologist and the transplant clinician is essential for the optimal care of these patients.

Pathologists also make important contributions in examining the patient's native heart to help clarify the etiology of the patient's heart failure. Examination of the failed allograft at the time of re-transplantation or autopsy may add to existing knowledge about the disease process. Pathologists are, in fact, in the perfect position to contribute to existing knowledge in the field of cardiac transplantation.

REFERENCES

1. Spiegelhalter DJ, Stovin PGI. An analysis of repeated biopsies following cardiac transplantation. Stat Med 1983;2:33–40.
2. Zerbe TR, Arena V. Diagnostic reliability of endomyocardial biopsy for assessment of cardiac allograft rejection. Hum Pathol 1988;19:1307–14.
3. Baraldi-Junkins C, Levin HR, Kasper EK, et al. Complications of endomyocardial biopsy in heart transplant patients. J Heart Lung Transplant 1993;12:63–7.
4. Pham MX, Teuteberg JJ, Kfoury AG, et al, for the IMAGE Study Group. Gene-expression profiling for rejection surveillance after cardiac transplantation. N Engl J Med 2010;362:1890–900.
5. Jarcho JA. Fear of rejection – monitoring the heart-transplant recipient. N Engl J Med 2010;362:1932–3.
6. Mehra MR, Parameshwar J. Gene expression profiling and cardiac allograft rejection monitoring: is IMAGE just a mirage? J Heart Lung Transplant 2010;29:599–602.
7. Hunt SA, Haddad F. The changing face of heart transplantation. J Am Coll Cardiol 2008;52:587–98.
8. Stewart S, Winters GL, Fishbein MC, et al. Revision of the 1990 working formulation for the standardization of nomenclature in the diagnosis of heart rejection. J Heart Lung Transplant 2005;24:1710–20.
9. Stone JR, Basso C, Baandrup UT, et al. Recommendations for processing cardiovascular surgical pathology specimens: a consensus statement from the Standards and Definitions Committee of the Society for Cardiovascular Pathology and the Association for European Cardiovascular Pathology. Cardiovasc Pathol 2012;21:2–16.
10. Spratt P, Sivathasan C, Macdonald P, et al. Role of endomyocardial biopsy to monitor late rejection after heart transplantation. J Heart Lung Transplant 1991;10:912–4.
11. White JA, Guiraudon C, Pflugfelder PW, et al. Routine surveillance myocardial biopsies are unnecessary beyond one year after heart transplantation. J Heart Lung Transplant 1995;14:1052–6.
12. Sethi GK, Kosaraju S, Arabia FA, et al. Is it necessary to perform surveillance endomyocardial biopsies in heart transplant recipients? J Heart Lung Transplant 1995;14:1047–51.
13. Heimansohn DA, Robison RJ, Paris JM 3rd, et al. Routine surveillance endomyocardial biopsy: late rejection after heart transplantation. Ann Thorac Surg 1997;64:1231–6.
14. Stehlik J, Starling RC, Movsesian MA, et al; Cardiac transplant Research Database Group. Utility of long-term surveillance endomyocardial biopsy: a multi-institutional analysis. J Heart Lung Transplant 2006;25:1402–9.

15. Kucirka LM, Maleszewski JJ, Segev DL, et al. Survey of North American pathologist practices regarding antibody-mediated rejection in cardiac transplant biopsies. Cardiovasc Pathol 2011;20:132–8.

16. Berry GJ, Angelini A, Burke MM, et al. The ISHLT working formulation for pathologic diagnosis of antibody-mediated rejection in heart transplantation: evolution and current status (2005-2011). J Heart Lung Transplant 2011;30:601–11.

17. Winters GL, Schoen FJ. Pathology of cardiac transplantation. In: Silver MD, Gotlieb AI, Schoen FJ, editors. Cardiovascular pathology. New York: Churchill Livingstone; 2001. p. 725–62.

18. Winters GL, Mitchell RM. The pathology of cardiac transplantation. In: McManus BM, Braunwald E, editors. Atlas of cardiovascular pathology. Philadelphia: Current Medicine Group LLC; 2008. p. 209–25.

19. Billingham ME, Cary NR, Hammond EH, et al. A working formulation for the standardization of nomenclature in the diagnosis of heart and lung rejection: heart rejection study group. J Heart Transplant 1990;9:587–93.

20. Yeoh TK, Frist WH, Eastburn TE, et al. Clinical significance of mild rejection of the cardiac allograft. Circulation 1992;86(Suppl 5):II267–71.

21. Lloveras JJ, Escourrou G, Delisle MB, et al. Evolution of untreated mild rejection in heart transplant recipients. J Heart Lung Transplant 1992;11:751–6.

22. Nielsen H, Sørensen FB, Nielsen B, et al. Reproducibility of the acute rejection diagnosis in human cardiac allografts. The Stanford classification and the International grading system. J Heart Lung Transplant 1993;12:239–43.

23. Rizeq MN, Masek MA, Billingham ME. Acute rejection: significance of elapsed time after transplantation. J Heart Lung Transplant 1994;13:862–8.

24. Fishbein MC, Bell G, Lones MA, et al. Grade 2 cellular heart rejection: does it exist? J Heart Lung Transplant 1994;13:1051–7.

25. Winters GL, Loh E, Schoen FJ. Natural history of focal moderate cardiac allograft rejection: is treatment warranted? Circulation 1995;91:1975–80.

26. Anguita M, López-Rubio F, Arizón JM, et al. Repetitive nontreated episodes of grade 1B or 2 acute rejection impair long-term cardiac graft function. J Heart Lung Transplant 1995;14:452–60.

27. Milano A, Caforio ALP, Livi U, et al. Evolution of focal moderate (International Society for Heart and Lung Transplantation Grade 2) rejection of the cardiac allograft. J Heart Lung Transplant 1996;15:456–60.

28. Brunner-La Rocca HP, Sütsch G, Schneider J, et al. Natural course of moderate cardiac allograft rejection (International Society for Heart Transplantation Grade 2) early and late after transplantation. Circulation 1996;94:1334–8.

29. Winters GL, McManus BM, Rapamycin Cardiac Rejection Treatment Trial Pathologists. Consistencies and controversies in the application of the ISHLT working formulation for cardiac transplant biopsy specimens. J Heart Lung Transplant 1996;15:728–35.

30. Winters GL. The challenge of endomyocardial biopsy interpretation in assessing cardiac allograft rejection. Curr Opin Cardiol 1997;12:146152.

31. Winters GL, Marboe CC, Billingham ME. The ISHLT grading system for cardiac transplant biopsies: clarification and commentary. J Heart Lung Transplant 1998;17:754–60.

32. Marboe CC, Billingham ME, Eisen H, et al. Nodular endocardial infiltrates (Quilty lesions) cause significant variability in diagnosis of ISHLT grade 2 and 3A rejection in cardiac allograft recipients. J Heart Lung Transplant 2005;24:S219–26.

33. Maleszewski JJ, Kucirka LM, Segev DL, et al. Survey of current practice related to grading of rejection in cardiac transplant recipients in North America. Cardiovasc Pathol 2011;20:261–5.

34. Hammond EH, Yowell RL, Nunoda S, et al. Vascular (humoral) rejection in heart transplantation: pathologic observations and clinical implications. J Heart Transplant 1989;8:430–43.

35. Hammond EH, Hansen JK, Spencer LS, et al. Vascular rejection in cardiac transplantation: histologic, immunopathologic, and ultrastructural features. Cardiovasc Pathol 1993;2:21–34.

36. Lones MA, Czer LS, Trento A, et al. Clinical-pathologic features of humoral rejection in cardiac allografts: a study in 81 consecutive patients. J Heart Lung Transplant 1995;14:151–62.

37. Michaels PJ, Espejo ML, Kobashigawa J, et al. Humoral rejection in cardiac transplantation: risk factors, hemodynamic consequences and relationship to transplant coronary artery disease. J Heart Lung Transplant 2003;22:58–69.

38. Kfoury AG, Renlund DG, Snow GL, et al. A clinical correlation study of severity of antibody-mediated rejection and cardiovascular mortality in heart transplantation. J Heart Lung Transplant 2009;28:51–7.

39. Wu GW, Kobashigawa JA, Fishbein MC, et al. Asymptomatic antibody-mediated rejection after heart transplantation predicts poor outcomes. J Heart Lung Transplant 2009;28:417–22.

40. Hammond EH, Stehlik J, Snow G, et al, and the Utah Transplant Affiliated Hospital (UTAH) Cardiac Transplant Program. Utility of histologic parameters in screening for antibody-mediated rejection of cardiac allograft: a study of 3,170 biopsies. J Heart Lung Transplant 2005;24:2015–21.

41. Fedrigo M, Gambino A, Benazzi E, et al. Role of morphologic parameters on endomyocardial biopsy to detect sub-clinical antibody-mediated rejection in heart transplantation. J Heart Lung Transplant 2011;30:1381–8.

42. Kobashigawa J, Crespo-Leiro M, Ensminger S, et al, on behalf of the Consensus Conference Participants. Report from a consensus conference on

antibody-mediated rejection in heart transplantation. J Heart Lung Transplant 2011;30:252–69.

43. Gries W, Farkas D, Winters GL, et al. Giant cell myocarditis: first report of disease recurrence in the transplanted heart. J Heart Lung Transplant 1992;11:370–4.

44. Oni AA, Hershberger RE, Norman DJ, et al. Recurrence of sarcoidosis in a cardiac allograft: control with augmented corticosteroids. J Heart Lung Transplant 1992;11:367–9.

45. Yager JE, Hernandez AF, Steenbergen C, et al. Recurrence of cardiac sarcoidosis in a heart transplant recipient. J Heart Lung Transplant 2005;24:1988–90.

46. Falk RH. Diagnosis and management of the cardiac amyloidoses. Circulation 2005;112:2047–60.

47. Kuppahally SS, Hunt SA, Valantine HA, et al. Recurrence of iron deposition in the cardiac allograft in a patient with non-HFE hemochromatosis. J Heart Lung Transplant 2006;25:144–7.

48. Moloney ED, Egan JJ, Kelly P, et al. Transplantation for myocarditis: a controversy revisited. J Heart Lung Transplant 2005;24:1103–10.

49. Gaudin PB, Rayburn BK, Hutchins GM, et al. Peritransplant injury to the myocardium associated with the development of accelerated arteriosclerosis in heart transplant recipients. Am J Surg Pathol 1994;18:338–46.

50. Fyfe B, Loh E, Winters GL, et al. Heart transplantation-associated perioperative ischemic myocardial injury: morphological features and clinical significance. Circulation 1996;93:1133–40.

51. Kottke-Marchant K, Ratliff NB. Endomyocardial lymphocytic infiltrates in cardiac transplant recipients. Arch Pathol Lab Med 1989;113:690–8.

52. Radio SJ, McManus BM, Winters GL, et al. Preferential endocardial residence of B-cells in the "Quilty effect" of human heart allografts: immunohistochemical distinction from rejection. Mod Pathol 1991;4:654–60.

53. Joshi A, Masek MA, Brown BW, et al. Quilty revisited: a 10-year perspective. Hum Pathol 1995;26:547–57.

54. Michaels PJ, Kobashigawa J, Laks H, et al. Differential expression of RANTES chemokine, TGF-β, and leukocyte phenotype in acute cellular rejection and Quilty B lesions. J Heart Lung Transplant 2001;20:407–16.

55. Chu KE, Ho EK, de la Torre L, et al. The relationship of nodular endocardial infiltrates (Quilty lesions) to survival, patient age, anti-HLA antibodies, and coronary artery disease following heart transplantation. Cardiovasc Pathol 2005;14:219–24.

56. Fishman JA. Infection in solid-organ transplant recipients. N Engl J Med 2007;357:2601–14.

57. Opelz G, Dohler B. Lymphomas after solid organ transplantation: a collaborative transplant study report. Am J Transplant 2003;4:222–30.

58. Eisen HJ, Hicks D, Kant JA, et al. Diagnosis of post-transplantation lymphoproliferative disorder by endomyocardial biopsy in a cardiac allograft recipient. J Heart Lung Transplant 1994;13:241–5.

59. Mitchell RN. Graft vascular disease: immune response meets the vessel wall. Annu Rev Pathol 2009;4:19–47.

60. Libby P, Pober JS. Chronic rejection. Immunity 2001; 14:387–97.

61. George JF, Pinderski LJ, Litovsky S, et al. Of mice and men: mouse models and the molecular mechanisms of post-transplant coronary artery disease. J Heart Lung Transplant 2005;24:2003–14.

62. Rahmani R, Cruz RP, Granville DJ, et al. Allograft vasculopathy versus atherosclerosis. Circ Res 2006;99:801–15.

63. Winters GL, Schoen FJ. Graft arteriosclerosis-induced myocardial pathology in heart transplant recipients: predictive value of endomyocardial biopsy. J Heart Lung Transplant 1997;16:985–93.

64. Karch SB, Billingham ME. Myocardial contraction bands revisited. Hum Pathol 1986;17:9–13.

65. Stehlik J, Edwards LB, Kucheryavaya AY, et al. The registry of the international society for heart and lung transplantation: twenty-eighth adult heart transplant report – 2011. J Heart Lung Transplant 2011; 30:1078–94.

DIAGNOSTIC BIOPSIES OF THE NATIVE HEART

James R. Stone, MD, PhD

KEYWORDS

- Endomyocardial biopsy • Amyloidosis • Myocarditis • Sarcoidosis • Hemochromatosis
- Fabry disease • Danon disease • Glycogen storage disease • Amiodarone toxicity
- Chloroquine toxicity

ABSTRACT

Endomyocardial biopsy in the nontransplant setting can be diagnostic for particular diseases. Such disorders include amyloidosis, myocarditis, sarcoidosis, iron overload, glycogen storage disorders, and lysosomal storage disorders. The diagnostic features of these disorders on endomyocardial biopsy will be discussed along with the impact of endomyocardial biopsy-based diagnoses on patient management and prognosis.

OVERVIEW OF NATIVE HEART BIOPSIES

Endomyocardial biopsy of native (nontransplanted) hearts can be a valuable diagnostic tool in some patients with cardiac dysfunction.[1]

Many common conditions do not show entirely diagnostic features on endomyocardial biopsy, including ischemic heart disease, hypertension, and many forms of inherited cardiomyopathies. In these settings, endomyocardial biopsy is still helpful in ruling out other conditions, some of which have specific treatments.

Conditions that can show diagnostic features on endomyocardial biopsy include amyloidosis, myocarditis, sarcoidosis, iron overload, glycogen storage disorders, and lysosomal storage disorders. The features of each of these conditions are described here.

Other conditions, including those that are less common or for which the histologic features on endomyocardial biopsy are less specific have been discussed elsewhere.[1]

In general, it is useful to stain all native endomyocardial biopsies with special stains that help to identify these conditions, and to perform electron microscopy when indicated.[2] In addition to hematoxylin and eosin (H&E) stained sections, our current approach is to stain all native endomyocardial biopsies with 6 special stains:

1. Masson trichrome
2. Congo red
3. periodic acid–Schiff (PAS)
4. PAS with diastase
5. Prussian blue
6. Luxol fast blue.

The precise staining protocol used for endomyocardial biopsies varies across different institutions.

CARDIAC AMYLOIDOSIS

OVERVIEW

The amyloidoses are a group of disorders characterized by the tissue deposition of abnormally folded protein possessing an extended beta-sheet conformation.[3] Cardiac amyloidosis is routinely definitively diagnosed by endomyocardial biopsy. At least 11 distinct types of amyloid are known to be deposited in the heart (Table 1).

MICROSCOPIC FEATURES OF CARDIAC AMYLOIDOSIS

In routine H&E-stained sections, amyloid deposits appear as extracellular eosinophilic amorphous material, and on Congo red stain, amyloid deposits have a salmon pink color (Fig. 1). Due to the ordered manner in which the Congo red dye binds to amyloid fibrils, Congo red staining enables

Department of Pathology, Massachusetts General Hospital, Harvard Medical School, Simches 8236, 185 Cambridge Street, Boston, MA 02114, USA
E-mail address: jrstone@partners.org

Surgical Pathology 5 (2012) 401–416
doi:10.1016/j.path.2012.04.004
1875-9181/12/$ – see front matter © 2012 Elsevier Inc. All rights reserved.

surgpath.theclinics.com

General Features
CARDIAC AMYLOIDOSIS

1. H&E Stain: Amorphorous extracellular eosionophilc material which does not show birefringence.

2. Congo Red Stain: Extracelluar material with salmon pink color and apple-green birefringence with plane-polarized light.

3. Electron Microscopy: Nonbranching overlapping fibrils.

4. A complete workup of cardiac amyloidosis includes establishing the type of amyloid present.

amyloid deposits to show birefringence. Unlike collagen, which is normally birefringent, amyloid is not birefringent with H&E staining, but shows apple-green birefringence with Congo red staining when using plane-polarized light. It should be noted that neither pink staining on Congo red-stained sections, or even apple-green birefringence on these slides with polarized light is diagnostic of amyloid. Congo red staining is diagnostic of amyloid when used in conjunction with H&E-stained slides to show that extracellular material lacking birefringence on H&E-stained slides, stains pink on Congo red-stained sections, and acquires apple-green birefringence with the Congo red stain. Other stains can be used to help identify amyloid deposits including trichrome, thioflavin-T and modified sulphated alcian blue, but these stains are not as specific for amyloid as is Congo red.

DIFFERENTIAL DIAGNOSIS OF CARDIAC AMYLOIDOSIS

In endomyocardial biopsies, the principle differential diagnosis for amyloid deposits is fibrosis or scar. The distinction between the two is usually readily established using the Congo red stain. In difficult cases, amyloid can be distinguished from fibrosis using electron microscopy, by which amyloid deposits show overlapping non-branching fibrils (Fig. 2). The differential diagnosis for amyloid also includes non-amyloid light-chain deposition disorder. While common in the kidney, this disorder is very uncommon in endomyocardial biopsies. Non-amyloid light-chain deposits will have a similar appearance to amyloid on H&E-stained sections but will not stain positively by Congo red. By electron microscopy, non-amyloid light-chain deposits appear as electron-dense granular deposits rather than the classic non-branching fibrils characteristic of amyloid (see Fig. 2).

SUBTYPING

Both prognosis and treatment of cardiac amyloidosis are dependent on the type of amyloid present.[4] Thus a complete workup of an endomyocardial biopsy

Table 1
Types of amyloid that involve the heart

Amyloid Subclass	Precursor Protein	Systemic vs Localized	Associations or Tissue Localization
AL	Immunoglobulin light chain	Systemic	Plasma cell neoplasm
AH	Immunoglobulin heavy chain	Systemic	Plasma cell neoplasm
ATTR	Transthyretin	Systemic	Senile systemic or hereditary
AA	Serum Amyloid A	Systemic	Chronic inflammation
$A\beta_2M$	β_2-microglobulin	Systemic	Hemodialysis
AApoAI	Apolipoprotein A-I	Systemic Localized	Hereditary Atherosclerotic plaques
AApoAII	Apolipoprotein A-II	Systemic	Hereditary
AApoAIV	Apolipoprotein A-IV	Systemic	Senile systemic
AGel	Gelsolin	Systemic	Hereditary
Abri	ABriPP	Systemic	Hereditary
AANF	Atrial natriuretic factor	Localized	Atria
—	unknown	Localized	Cardiac valves, mural thrombi

Adapted from Collins AB, Smith RN, Stone JR. Classification of amyloid deposits in diagnostic cardiac specimens by immunofluorescence. Cardiovasc Pathol 2009;18:205–16.

Fig. 1. Cardiac amyloid-osis. (*A*) H&E stained section at 400× magnifica-tion showing amorphous eosinophilic interstitial material, which could be misinterpreted as fibrosis. (*B*) Congo red stained sec-tion of the same case at 400× magnification showing the typical salmon pink color of amyloid.

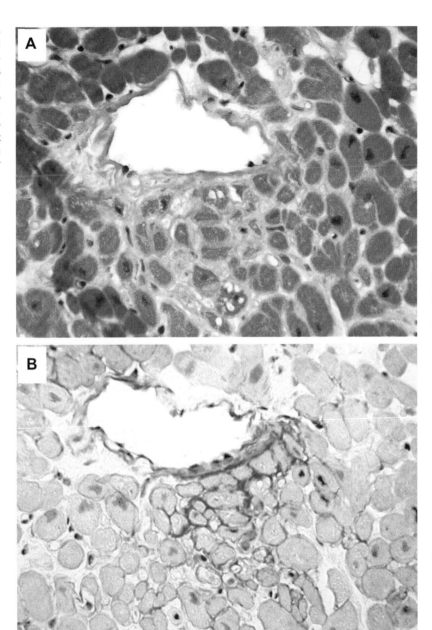

containing amyloid includes subtyping of the amyloid (Fig. 3). Potential methods to subtype amyloid in-clude immunohistochemistry, immunofluorescence, immuno-electron microscopy, immunoblotting, pro-tein sequencing, and mass spectrometry.[5–9] Immu-nohistochemistry is the most widely available technique, but is also the least reliable, with this approach prone to misclassification of the amyloid.[5]

Immunofluorescence, which requires fresh frozen tissue, appears to have good sensitivity and speci-ficity for AL and AA amyloid, but probably has less sensitivity for ATTR amyloid. All antibody-based approaches to amyloid subtyping should be per-formed with a panel of antibodies, with appropriate positive controls. Mass spectrometry-based amyloid subtyping can be performed on paraffin-embedded

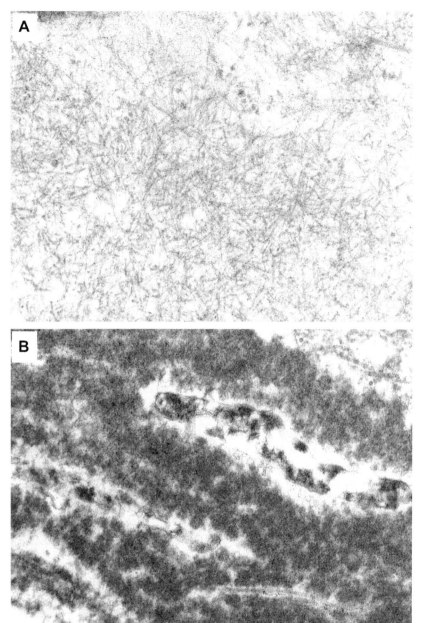

Fig. 2. Electron microscopy of immunoglobulin-related deposition diseases in the heart. (*A*) Transmission electron micrograph at 34,000× magnification showing nonbranching overlapping fibrils characteristic of amyloid. (*B*) Transmission electron micrograph at 45,000× magnification showing dense granular deposits indicative of non-amyloid light-chain deposition disease.

material, but is currently only performed in approved clinical diagnostic laboratories in a few centers.

PROGNOSIS IN CARDIAC AMYLOIDOSIS

Patients with AL cardiac amyloidosis and heart failure have a median survival of only 4 to 6 months without treatment, while patients with cardiac involvement by senile systemic amyloidosis and inherited transthyretin amyloidoses have a median survival of 5 to 6 years.[10–12] In cardiac AL amyloidosis patients, chemotherapy with or without autologous stem cell rescue allows for an overall median survival of 1 to 3 years. In patients with heart failure due to cardiac AL amyloidosis, the toxic effects of standard chemotherapy for plasma

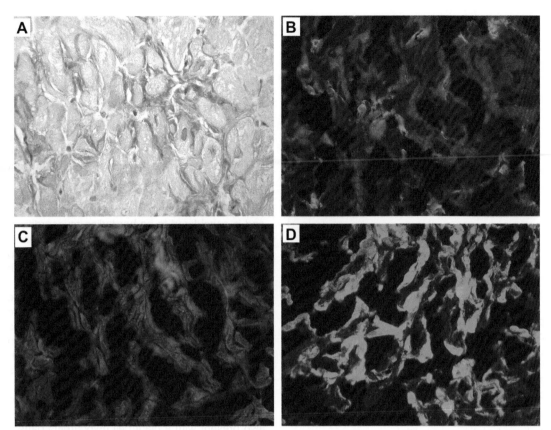

Fig. 3. Subtyping cardiac amyloid. (*A*) Congo red stained section at 400x magnification showing interstitial amyloid deposition. Immunofluorescence on fresh-frozen tissue for kappa light chain (*B*), lambda light chain (*C*) and transthyretin (*D*) showing specific staining of the amyloid for transthyretin, indicating the presence of ATTR amyloidosis.

cell neoplasms limit its utility. However, most patients in heart failure with AL cardiac amyloidosis who first undergo cardiac transplantation before chemotherapy and autologous stem cell transplantation survive more than 4 years.[13]

Pitfalls
DIAGNOSIS OF
CARDIAC AMYLOIDOSIS

! Amyloid can be easily missed on routine H&E-stained slides.

! Not everything that stains with Congo red is amyloid.

! Subtyping amyloid with antibody-based approaches requires a panel of antibodies.

! Use of immunohistochemistry on paraffin-embedded tissue can result in misclassification of the amyloid subtype.

MYOCARDITIS

OVERVIEW

Myocarditis is a condition in which inflammation infiltrates the myocardium. Myocarditis may be due to infections, autoimmune diseases, reactions to drugs or environmental stimuli, or may be largely idiopathic.

This discussion focuses on myocarditis that is either idiopathic or secondary to viral infections, autoimmune diseases, or reactions to drugs and environmental stimuli, and does not specifically address myocarditis due to bacterial, fungal, and parasitic infections of the heart.

Patients with myocarditis may present with a variety of signs and symptoms including chest pain, heart failure, palpitations, syncope, or sudden death. Definitive diagnosis often requires endomyocardial biopsy. Myocarditis may be focal, multifocal or diffuse with endomyocardial biopsy often showing poor sensitivity for the former two

General Features
MYOCARDITIS

1. There is an inflammatory infiltrate which cannot be attributed to a more routine process such as ischemic heart disease.

2. Myocardial injury is present in most types of myocarditis.

3. The pathologic classification of myocarditis is primarily based on the composition and extent of the inflammatory infiltrate and the degree of myocardial injury.

4. Treatment and prognosis are dependent on the type of myocarditis present.

patterns, but good sensitivity for the diffuse pattern. It is best for the endomyocardial biopsy to contain four or more fragments of myocardium when assessing for myocarditis. Myocarditis is subclassified histologically based on the pattern of inflammatory cell infiltration. There are four principal subtypes:

1. Lymphocytic myocarditis
2. Giant cell myocarditis
3. Hypersensitivity myocarditis
4. Acute necrotizing eosinophilic myocarditis.

Their key histologic features and associations are listed in Table 2. Note that drug reactions are most commonly associated with hypersensitivity myocarditis, but have been linked will all four histologic patterns of myocarditis.

MICROSCOPIC FEATURES OF MYOCARDITIS

The key histologic feature of myocarditis is the presence of inflammation, which cannot be attributed to another routine process such as ischemic heart disease. In lymphocytic myocarditis, the inflammatory infiltrate is lymphocyte predominant (Fig. 4). By Dallas Criteria, myocyte injury should also be present on endomyocardial biopsy, otherwise the biopsy is not diagnostic for myocarditis and is considered to be borderline myocarditis.[14] It should be remembered that endomyocardial biopsies of normal myocardium may contain up to 4 to 5 lymphocytes per 0.16 mm^2 400x high power field.[15]

Giant cell myocarditis is characterized by the presence of giant cells within a lymphohistiocytic inflammatory background, which often includes occasional eosinophils.[16] The giant cells are often found at the leading edge of the inflammatory infiltrates bordering live myocytes (Fig. 5). There is often extensive myocyte injury. Giant cell myocarditis is typically an idiopathic condition limited to the heart. In rare occasions, drug reactions can also present with a giant cell myocarditis pattern of inflammatory response.[17] Giant cell myocarditis may also be part of a systemic giant cell polymyositis occurring as a paraneoplastic phenomenon in patients with thymoma.[18]

Hypersensitivity myocarditis is normally characterized by the presence of eosinophils and

Table 2
Histologic subclassificaiton of myocarditis

Subtype	Key Histologic Features	Associations
Lymphocytic myocarditis	Lymphoctye predominant inflammation with myocyte injury	Idiopathic, viral infections, autoimmue diseases, drug reactions
Giant cell myocaritis	Giant cells with extensive acute myocyte injury, occasional eosinophils	Idiopathic, drug reactions, thymoma
Hypersensitivity myocarditis	Eosionphils and macrophages, with variable myocyte injury May be lymphocyte predominant May contain giant cells	Drug reactions, chronic infections, idiopathic
Acute necrotizing eosinophilic myocarditis	Dense eosionphilc infiltrates with extensive myocyte injury May contain giant cells	Idiopathic, drug reactions

Fig. 4. Lymphocytic myocarditis. The H&E-stained section at 400× magnification shows a dense lymphocytic infiltrate associated with myocyte injury.

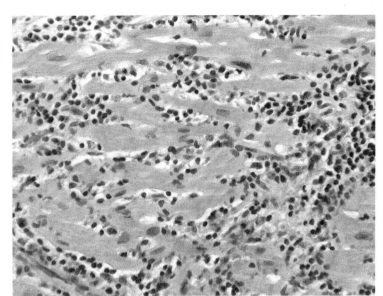

Fig. 5. Giant cell myocarditis. There is a dense inflammatory infiltrate containing giant cells with scattered eosinophils in a region with myocyte injury. H&E-stained section at 400× magnification.

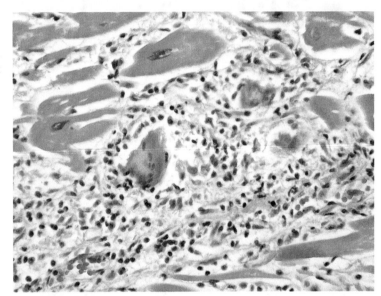

Fig. 6. Hypersensitivity myocarditis. The H&E-stained section at 600x magnification shows an interstitial infiltration by eosinophils without overt myocyte injury.

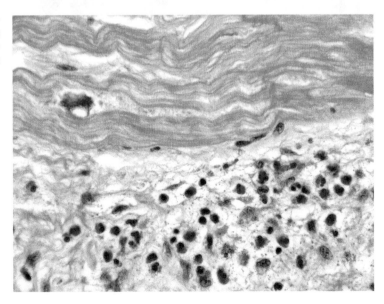

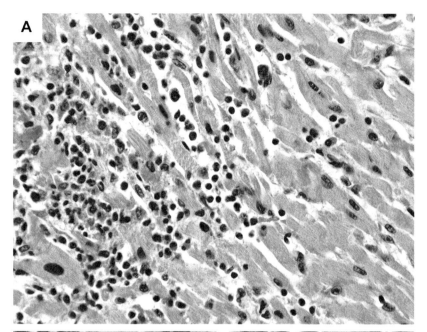

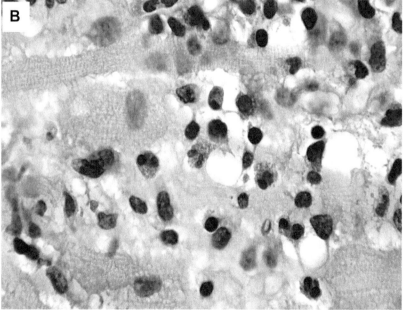

Fig. 7. Acute necrotizing eosinophilic myocarditis (ANEM). (*A*) There is a necrotizing inflammatory infiltrate associated with myocyte injury (400× magnification). (*B*) The infiltrate contains numerous eosinophils (1000× magnification).

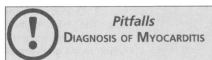

macrophages (**Fig. 6**).[19] Some cases may be lymphocyte predominant, and granulomatous inflammation may be present. The amount of myocyte injury is variable, with many cases showing little to no myocyte injury and some cases showing more extensive injury. In the more severe cases of hypersensitivity myocarditis, the histology borders with that of acute necrotizing eosinophilic myocarditis (ANEM), which may simply be an extreme form of hypersensitivity myocarditis.[20,21] In ANEM there is extensive myocyte injury associated with eosinophilic inflammatory infiltrates, which also contain macrophages and lymphocytes (**Fig. 7**). Giant cells can be present in ANEM, but are typically located within areas of necrosis ingesting necrotic myocytes.

DIFFERENTIAL DIAGNOSIS OF MYOCARDITIS

It is important to distinguish active myocarditis from healing myocardial injury due to other causes, such as ischemia and catecholamine toxicity. In general, in myocarditis the inflammatory infiltrate should be seen around live cells, and in most cases attacking and injuring the live cells. In contrast, granulation tissue and a neutrophilic or mixed inflammatory infiltrate associated primarily with necrotic cells are both more consistent with healing injury. In cases with extensive necrosis as may be present in giant cell myocarditis and ANEM, the presence of bacterial and fungal myocarditis can be assessed with special stains for microorganisms. Myocarditis should also be distinguished from sarcoidosis, discussed below.

ANCILLARY STUDIES FOR MYOCARDITIS

Immunohistochemistry can be helpful to define the numbers of the specific cell types present: CD3 for T-lymphocytes, CD20 for B-lymphocytes and CD68 for macrophages. Since lymphocytic myocarditis is in some cases associated with viral infections, there has been interest in some centers in performing molecular analyses for viral genomes in endomyocardial biopsy specimens. The viruses often sought include adenovirus, enterovirus, human herpes virus 6, influenza viruses A and B, parvovirus B19, and rhinovirus. Currently there is much controversy concerning the utility of such viral molecular studies.[2]

PROGNOSIS IN MYOCARDITIS

Prognosis in myocarditis is dependent on the type of myocarditis present. Patients with biopsy-proven lymphocytic myocarditis have a 5-year survival of approximately 50%, which contrasts to patients with borderline myocarditis, who have a 5-year survival of more than 80%.[22] For patients with giant cell myocarditis, the average survival is only about 3 months without treatment and about 12 months with aggressive immunosuppressive therapy.[23] However, the majority of patients with giant cell myocarditis who undergo cardiac transplantation survive more than 5 years.[24] Hypersensitivity myocarditis can be self-limited, if the offending agent is identified and avoided before sudden cardiac death. However in ANEM, more than half of the patients die within a few days.[21]

SARCOIDOSIS

OVERVIEW

Sarcoidosis is a systemic disease characterized by the infiltration of tissue by granuomatous inflammation. The underlying etiology remains unclear. In a large autopsy study, 27% of patients with sarcoidosis had cardiac involvement.[25] Patients with cardiac involvement by sarcoidosis may present with unexplained cardiac dysrhythmias or heart failure. Due to the focal nature of the disease, endomyocardial biopsy is only positive in around 19% to 25% of patients with presumed cardiac saroidosis.[26,27]

MICROSCOPIC FEATURES OF SARCOIDOSIS

Cardiac sarcoidosis is characterized by the presence of granulomatous inflammation, which may include both compact non-necrotizing granulomas and giant cells (**Fig. 8**). Fibrosis is common, but actual myocyte necrosis is typically absent or

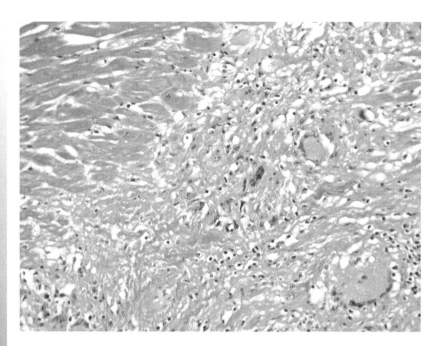

Fig. 8. Cardiac sarcoidosis. The H&E stained section at 200× magnification shows granulomatous inflammation with giant cells and extensive scarring, but no acute myocyte necrosis.

sparse. An accompanying lymphocytic infiltrate composed primarily of T-cells is usually present. Plasma cells and eosinophils may be present, but are usually not conspicuous.

DIFFERENTIAL DIAGNOSIS OF SARCOIDOSIS

An import issue is to differentiaate sarcoidosis from giant cell myocarditis and in some cases lymphocytic myocarditis.

In giant cell myocarditis there will be a more mixed inflammatory infiltrate, with more plasma cells and eosinophils than are typically present in sarcoidosis. In addition, compact granulomas are typically not present in giant cell myocarditis.

Both giant cell myocarditis and lymphocytic myocarditis often show more acute myocardial injury than is present in sarcoidosis.

Borderline lymphocytic myocarditis may in some patients represent the lymphocytic component of sarcoidosis in which the granulomatous component was not present on the biopsy.

In sarcoidosis there is often more scarring than typically pressent in the early stages of giant cell myocarditis or active lymphocytic myocarditis. However, distinguishing chronic endstage giant cell myocarditis from sarcoidosis may be difficult.

Hypersensitivity myocarditis, which may contain granulomatous inflammation, typically shows more eosinophils and less scarring than occur in sarcoidosis. Necrotizing granulomas are more indicative of infectious disases than sarcoidosis. In addition, special stains for microorganisms are helpful to rule out infectious diseases, particularly fungal and mycobacterial infections.

PROGNOSIS IN SARCOIDOSIS

In general, patients with sarcoidosis have a good survival rate. Even patients with stage IV pulmonary involvement have a 10-year survival of over 80%[28]; however, approximately one-third of patients with cardiac sarcoidosis die within 3 years of presentation.[26]

IRON OVERLOAD

Iron overload occurs in the heart both as a consequence of inherited disorders of iron metabolism such as hemochromatosis, and secondarily as a consequence of multiple transfusions.[29–31] On H&E-stained sections, the iron appears as brown granular material within the myocytes (**Fig. 9**), and can be confused with routine lipofuscin. However, iron deposits are not as restricted to perinuclear areas as is lipofuscin. On Prussian blue stain, the iron deposits acquire a blue color. Any iron present within cardiac myocytes observed on Prussian blue stain is considered abnormal. Iron is seen routinely in macrophages in areas of healing myocardial injury in numerous conditions. Primary genetic

Fig. 9. Cardiac iron overload. Shown is an endomyocardial biopsy from a patient with hemochromatosis. (A) On H&E stain the myocytes are vacuolated and contain excessive brown pigment. (B) On Prussian blue stain there is extensive positive staining for iron within the cardiac myocytes.

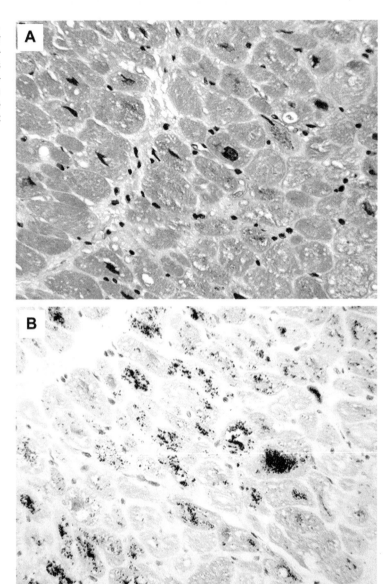

Fig. 10. Cardiac glycogen storage disorder. The H&E stained section at 400× magnification shows vacuolization of the myocytes with material present within the vacuoles. See also Figs. 11 and 12.

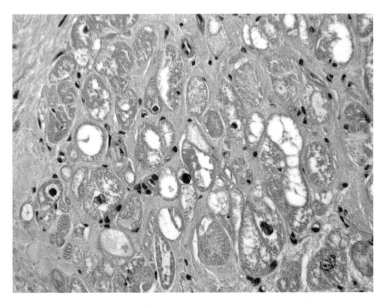

and secondary forms of iron overload cannot be distinguished on endomyocardial biopsy.

GLYCOGEN STORAGE DISORDERS

Glycogen storage diseases include inherited disorders such as alpha-glucosidase deficiency (Pompe disease), mutations of the LAMP2 gene (Danon disease), and mutations of PRKAG2.[32–34]

Histologically the myocardium often shows extensive and diffuse vacuolization with material in the vacuoles (Fig. 10). The material in the vacuoles stains red on PAS stain, but negatively on PAS with diastase digestion (Fig. 11). Electron microscopy will confirm the material to be glycogen and will demonstrate if the excess glycogen is within membrane-bound structures (Fig. 12). The glycogen is predominantly

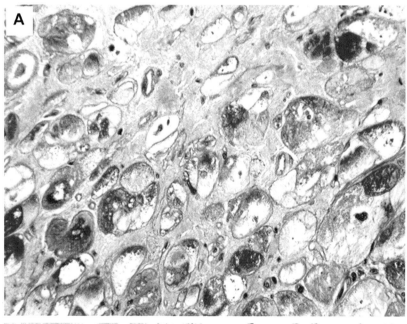

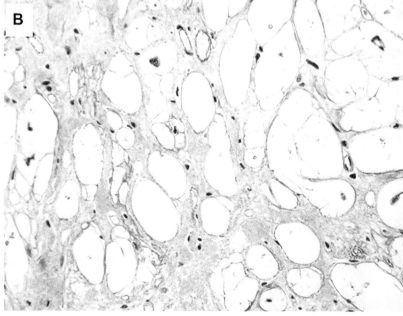

Fig. 11. Glycogen storage disorder. (A) PAS stain of the case in Fig. 10 shows the material present within the vacuoles to stain bright red. However, staining with PAS after diastase digestion shows no staining of the material (B), indicating the material within the vacuoles to be glycogen.

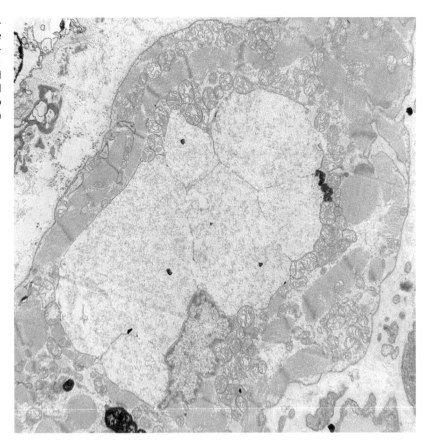

Fig. 12. Electron microscopy of glycogen storage disorder. Transmission electron microscopy at 4,500× magnification, performed on the case in **Figs. 10** and **11** reveals the material to be glycogen that is within membrane-bound structures.

membrane bound is some glycogen storage disorders such as Pompe disease and Danon disease, but is predominantly not membrane bound in other disorders, such as mutations of PRKAG2. Danon disease may also show lamellar inclusions as found in lysosomal storage disorders. It is often not possible to subtype the precise form of glycogen storage disease present from histologic assessment of an endomyocardial biopsy. However the definitive identification of a glycogen storage disease helps to focus subsequent genetic testing.

LYSOSOMAL STORAGE DISORDERS

Lysosomal storage disorders include inherited conditions such as Fabry disease as well as side effects and toxicities of medications including amiodarone, chloroquine, and hydroxychloroquine.[35–39] Histologically the myocardium will typically deomonstrate extensive vacuolization with material present within the vacuoles (**Fig. 13**). In many cases, the material within the vacuoles will stain blue on luxol fast blue/H&E stain, in contrast to lipofuscin, which normally remains brown or may stain light green. Electron microscopy is necessary to confirm the diagnosis, and will typically demonstrate lamellar inclusions within the cardiac myoctyes (**Fig. 14**). In chloroqine/hydroxychloroquine toxicity, there may also be excess glycogen and curvilinear bodies present on electron microscopy.[38,39] It is often not possible to definitvely subclassify the type of lysosmal storage disorder present based on the histologic assessment of an endomyocardial biopsy. However, the definitive identification of a lysosomal storage disorder helps to focus the clinical investigation.

414

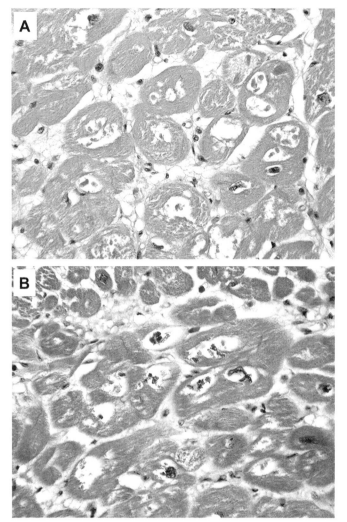

Fig. 13. Cardiac lysosomal storage disorder. (A) On an H&E-stained section at 400× magnification, the cardiac myocytes appear vacuolated with material within the vacuoles. (B) On Luxol fast blue/H&E stain at 400× magnification, the material within the vacuoles stains bright blue indicating a lysosomal storage disorder.

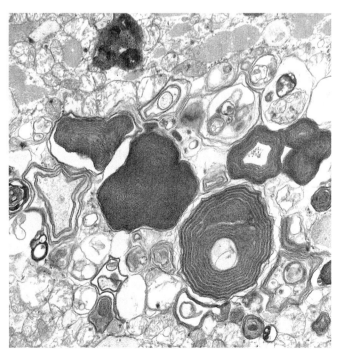

Fig. 14. Amiodarone toxicity. Shown is a transmission electron micrograph at 9,100× magnification from a patient with amiodarone toxicity. There are numerous dense lamellar inclusions indicative of a lysosomal storage disorder.

REFERENCES

1. Leone O, Veinot JP, Angelini A, et al. Consensus statement on endomyocardial biopsy from the European Association for Cardiovascular Pathology and the Society for Cardiovascular Pathology 2011. Cardiovasc Pathol, in press.

2. Stone JR, Basso C, Baandrup UT, et al. Recommendations for processing cardiovascular surgical pathology specimens: a consensus statement from the Standards and Definitions Committee of the Society for Cardiovascular Pathology and the Association for European Cardiovascular Pathology. Cardiovasc Pathol 2012;21:2–16.

3. Merlini G, Bellotti V. Molecular mechanisms of amyloidosis. N Engl J Med 2003;349:583–96.

4. Falk RH. Diagnosis and management of the cardiac amyloidoses. Circulation 2005;112:2047–60.

5. Collins AB, Smith RN, Stone JR. Classification of amyloid deposits in diagnostic cardiac specimens by immunofluorescence. Cardiovasc Pathol 2009; 18:205–16.

6. Crotty TB, Li CY, Edwards WD, et al. Amyloidosis and endomyocardial biopsy: correlation of extent and pattern of deposition with amyloid immunophenotype in 100 cases. Cardiovasc Pathol 1995;4:39–42.

7. Arbustini E, Morbini P, Verga L, et al. Light and electron microscopy immunohistochemical characterization of amyloid deposits. Amyloid 1997;4:157–70.

8. Benson MD, Breall J, Cummings OW, et al. Biochemical characterization of amyloid by endomyocardial biopsy. Amyloid 2009;16:9–14.

9. Vrana JA, Gamez JD, Madden BJ, et al. Classification of amyloidosis by laser microdissection and mass spectrometry-based proteomic analysis in clinical biopsy specimens. Blood 2009;114:4957–9.

10. Falk RH, Dubrey SW. Amyloid heart disease. Prog Cardiovasc Dis 2010;52:347–61.

11. Rapezzi C, Merlini G, Quarta CC, et al. Systemic cardiac amyloidoses: disease profiles and clinical courses of the 3 main types. Circulation 2009;120: 1203–12.

12. Skinner M, Sanchorawala V, Seldin DC, et al. High-dose melphalan and autologous stem-cell transplantation in patients with AL amyloidosis: an 8-year study. Ann Intern Med 2004;140:85–93.

13. Dey BR, Chung SS, Spitzer TR, et al. Cardiac transplantation followed by dose-intensive melphalan and autologous stem-cell transplantation for light chain amyloidosis and heart failure. Transplantation 2010;90:905–11.

14. Aretz HT, Billingham ME, Edwards WD, et al. Myocarditis: a histopathologic definition and classification. Am J Cardiovasc Pathol 1987;1:3–14.

15. Linder J, Cassling RS, Rogler WC, et al. Immunohistochemical characterization of lymphocytes in uninflamed ventricular myocardium: implications for myocarditis. Arch Pathol Lab Med 1985;109: 917–20.

16. Cooper LT, Berry GJ, Rizeq M, et al. Giant cell myocarditis. J Heart Lung Transplant 1995;14: 394–401.

17. Daniels PR, Berry GJ, Tazelaar HD, et al. Giant cell myocarditis as a manifestation of drug hypersensitivity. Cardiovasc Pathol 2000;9:287–91.

18. Venna N, Gonzalez RG, Zukerberg LR. A woman in her 90s with unilateral ptosis. N Engl J Med 2011; 365:2413–22.

19. Fenoglio JJ, McAllister HA, Mullick FG. Drug related myocarditis: 1. hypersensitivity myocarditis. Hum Pathol 1981;12:900–7.

20. Getz MA, Subramanian R, Logemann T, et al. Acute necrotizing eosinophilic myocarditis as a manifestation of severe hypersensitivity myocarditis. Ann Intern Med 1991;115:201–2.

21. Sabatine MS, Poh KK, Mega JL, et al. A 31-year-old woman with rash, fever, and hypotension. N Engl J Med 2007;357:2167–78.

22. Magnani JW, Danik HJ, Dec GW, et al. Survival in biopsy-proven myocarditis: a long-term retrospective analysis of the histopathologic, clinical, and hemodynamic predictors. Am Heart J 2006;151: 463–70.

23. Cooper LT, Berry GJ, Shabetai R. Idiopathic giant-cell myocarditis - natural history and treatment. N Engl J Med 1997;336:1860–6.

24. Cooper LT. Giant cell myocarditis: diagnosis and treatment. Herz 2000;25:291–8.

25. Silverman KJ, Hutchins GM, Bulkley BH. Cardiac sarcoid: a clinicopathologic study of 84 unselected patients with systemic sarcoidosis. Circulation 1978;58:1204–11.

26. Uemura A, Morimoto S, Hiramitsu S, et al. Histologic diagnostic rate of cardiac sarcoidosis: evaluation of endomyocardial biopsies. Am Heart J 1999;138: 299–302.

27. Ardehali H, Howard DL, Hariri A, et al. A positive endomyocardial biopsy result for sarcoid is associated with poor prognosis in patients with initially unexplained cardiomyopathy. Am Heart J 2005;150: 459–63.

28. Nardi A, Brillet PY, Letoumelin P, et al. Stage IV sarcoidosis: comparison of survival with the general population and causes of death. Eur Respir J 2011; 38:1368–73.

29. Olson LJ, Edwards WD, McCall JT, et al. Cardiac iron deposition in idiopathic hemochromatosis: histologic and analytic assessment of 14 hearts from autopsy. J Am Coll Cardiol 1987;10:1239–43.

30. Pietrangelo A. Hereditary hemochromatosis - a new look at an old disease. N Engl J Med 2004;350: 2383–97.

31. Lombardo T, Tamburino C, Bartoloni G, et al. Cardiac iron overload in thalassemic patients: an endomyocardial biopsy study. Ann Hematol 1995;71: 135–41.

32. Ben-Ami R, Puglisi J, Haider T, et al. The Mount Sinai Hospital clinicalpathological conference: a 45-year-old man with Pompe's disease and dilated cardiomyopathy. Mt Sinai J Med 2001;68:205–12.

33. Burwinkel B, Scott JW, Buhrer C, et al. Fatal congenital heart glycogenosis caused by a recurrent activating R531Q mutation in the gamma-2-subunit of AMP-activated protein kinase (PRKAG2), not by phosphorylase kinase deficiency. Am J Hum Genet 2005;76:1034–49.

34. Balmer C, Ballhausen D, Bosshard NU, et al. Familial X-linked cardiomyopathy (Danon disease): diagnostic confirmation by mutation analysis of the LAMP2 gene. Eur J Pediatr 2005;164:509–14.

35. Thurberg BL, Fallon JT, Mitchell R, et al. Cardiac microvascular pathology in Fabry disease: evaluation of endomyocardial biopsies before and after enzyme replacement therapy. Circulation 2009;119: 2561–7.

36. Staretz-Chacham O, Lang TC, LaMarca ME, et al. Lysosomal storage disorders in the newborn. Pediatrics 2009;123:1191–207.

37. Arbustini E, Grasso M, Salerno JA, et al. Endomyocardial biopsy finding in two patients with idiopathic dilated cardiomyopathy receiving long-term treatment with amiodarone. Am J Cardiol 1991;67:661–2.

38. Newton-Cheh C, Lin AE, Baggish AL, et al. A 47-year-old man with systemic lupus erythematosus and heart failure. N Engl J Med 2011;364:1450–60.

39. August C, Holzhausen HJ, Schmoldt A, et al. Histological and ultrastructural findings in chloroquine-induced cardiomyopathy. J Mol Med 1995;73:73–7.

PATHOLOGY OF THE AORTA

Marc Halushka, MD, PhD

KEYWORDS

• Aorta • Aneurysm • Dissection • Marfan syndrome

ABSTRACT

The aorta is a distinctive surgical pathology specimen removed most frequently for aneurysm or dissection. Genetic syndromes, inflammatory processes and acquired diseases of aging result in aortic pathology; these are presented in terms of pathology, differential diagnosis and classification schemes. The pathologic context of a variety of commonly encountered histopathologies is described.

Key Features
GROSS AORTIC PATHOLOGY

1. The presence of dissecting blood in the media or adventitia.

2. Tree-barking

3. Atherosclerotic plaques

4. Cross-sectional diameter

OVERVIEW OF THE AORTA

The aorta is a rare, but still frequently encountered, surgical pathology specimen. Generally, when it is removed, it is done for cause (aneurysm, infection, dissection, tumor) and the surgery is considered to be the definitive treatment. Fortunately, for the pathologist, this means that there is often no need make a novel diagnosis on their limited specimens. But, there are a few histologic appearances that should be conveyed to the surgeon or clinician that can change patient management. Therefore, proper grossing and evaluation of this specimen are important. This article provides information on handling and diagnostic tools for the aorta and highlight diagnoses that are or are not critical to the care of the patient.

GROSSING CONSIDERATIONS FOR THE AORTA

All resected aortic specimens should be handled with the same approach. The specimen may arrive either as an intact segment of aorta or in fragments.

- If intact, it should be measured for diameter and height.
- The overall shape, which should be noted, can also suggest the aneurysm type.
- If in fragments, the entirety of the pieces *in toto* should be recorded.
- Coloration and wall thickness should be recorded.
- If a tumor is suspected, the superior, inferior and adventitial margins can be inked.
- Sections should be taken as ~2.5 cm segments of aorta that are in the circumferential plane (perpendicular to blood flow).
- A minimum of six sections should be taken for histology, capturing any obvious gross pathology and processed on their cut sides to evaluate the full thickness of the wall.
- In addition to H&E staining, I recommend an elastic stain (ex. Movat, Miller's, or VVG) for all aortic specimens, however that is not a common practice at many institutions.[1,2]

In summary, a normal aortic specimen should be processed into six segments (usually across

Department of Pathology, Johns Hopkins University School of Medicine, 720 Rutland Avenue, Ross Building, Room 632L, Baltimore, MD 21205, USA

E-mail address: mhalush1@jhmi.edu

Surgical Pathology 5 (2012) 417–433
doi:10.1016/j.path.2012.04.005

two cassettes) and have both H&E and elastic stains requested for initial evaluation (Fig. 1).

GENERAL GROSS FEATURES OF THE AORTA

Gross features of the aorta are generally applicable to all specimens and will be covered together here. In all cases removed for aneurysm, attention must be given to describe any areas of dissection. An active dissection may appear as red to black material within the outer media or adventitia of the aorta (Fig. 2). Tree barking is a gross feature notable for wrinkles, plaques, and ridges in the intimal wall associated with patchy thickening.[3] Tree barking is a feature of an inflammatory aortitis (eg, syphilis, Takayasu arteritis), but it is not usually a genetic cause of aortic disease (eg, Marfan syndrome, Turner syndrome).[4] Generally, older individuals undergoing aortic surgery have atherosclerotic plaque formation that should be characterized. Atherosclerotic plaques are intimally-based lesions that are firm, raised areas measuring up to several centimeters in diameter and can be ulcerated, hemorrhagic and/or calcified.

Key Features
HISTOLOGIC AORTIC PATHOLOGY

1. Inflammation. Seen in giant cell aortitis, Takayasu arteritis, infectious aortitis, lymphoplasmacytic aortitis and IgG4-RD aortitis.

2. Medial degeneration. Seen in genetic diseases such as Marfan Syndrome, Turner Syndrome, Arterial-Toruosity Syndrome and others.

3. Laminar medial necrosis. Seen in a variety of aortic aneurismal diseases, predominantly among older individuals.

They range in color from tan to yellow to red and often are easily disrupted during manipulation.[5] Younger individuals who require aortic surgery for aneurysm often have grossly unremarkable aortas. Additional specific gross findings – coarctation and tumor are described within their own entities below.

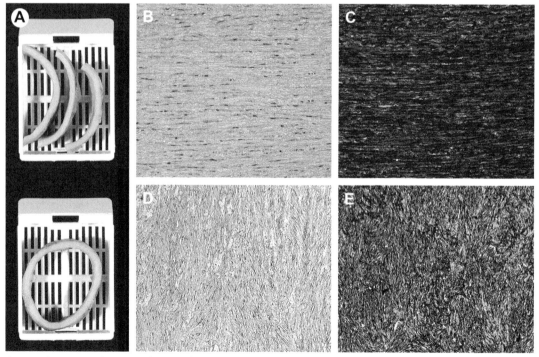

Fig. 1. Orientation of tissue and proper histology. (A) Pieces of aorta should be cut perpendicular to the direction of flow and placed on edge for proper histology. (B, C) Normal appearing aorta media with typical lamellar units, smooth muscle cell nuclei organized/dense elastic fibers as seen by H&E and Movat Pentachrome. (D, E) Improperly oriented aorta tissue which is suboptimal for diagnostic purposes. The lamellar units are not discernable and the elastic stain gives a highly irregular appearance despite it being a normal aorta (H&E and Movat Pentachrome).

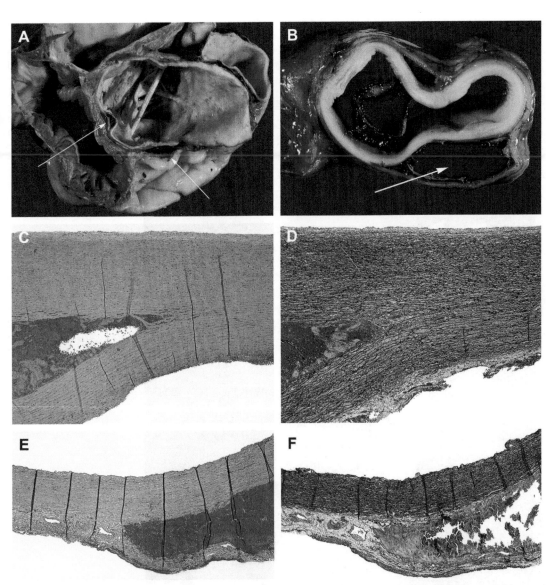

Fig. 2. Presentations of aneurysms. (*A*) A gross image of dark-staining blood trapped within the medial layer of the ascending aorta (*white arrows*) in a case of bicuspid aortic valve and aneurysm. (*B*) Cross-sectional view of a segment of ascending aorta with atherosclerotic plaques (yellow/white intimal lesions) and a dissection noted by a collection of blood (*white arrow*) in the outer medial layer. (*C*) Histologic view of a medial dissection (H&E). (*D*) Often the blood dissects through histologically normal lamellae as noted by the normal elastic fiber organization (Movat Pentachrome). (*E, F*) Histologic view of an adventitial dissection. The blood is outside the media, being trapped only by the dense connective tissue of the adventitia (H&E and Movat Pentachrome).

ANEURYSM TYPES

Aneurysms generally are fusiform (diffuse) or saccular (outpouchings) (**Fig. 3**).

Diffuse aneurysms are the most typical form seen in the ascending aorta and can have cylindrical or globular expansions. They are a concentric expansion of the aortic wall diameter. These aneurysms can appear anywhere from the aortic root, along the ascending aorta, through the aortic arch and more rarely along the descending aorta. Aneurysms of the aortic root can cause aortic valve regurgitation as the valve leaflets are no longer able to extend across the luminal diameter.

Saccular aneurysms are the result of a localized weakness on one side of the vessel wall leading to expansion and thinning of that area. Berry aneurysms along the circle of Willis are prototypical

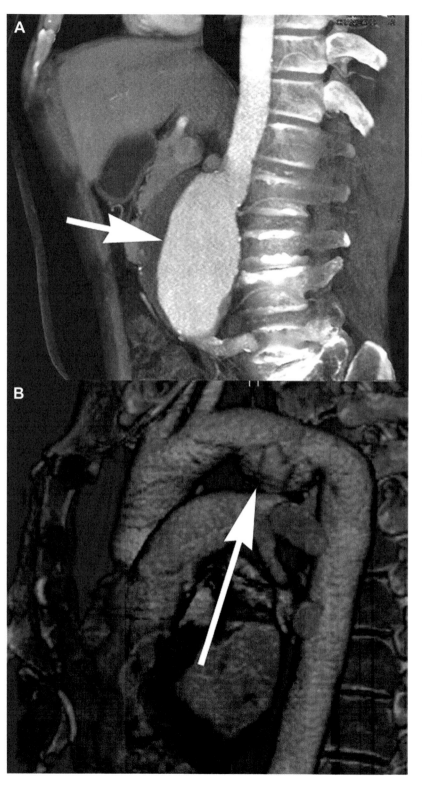

Fig. 3. Imaging of aortic aneurysms. (A) A fusiform aneurysm of the abdominal aorta is noted by its concentric dilatation (white arrow) by CT scan. (B) There is a saccular aneurysm of the transverse/distal aorta in this vascular 3D-reconstruction. (Images courtesy of Dr James Black.)

for this type of aneurysm. In the aorta, saccular aneurysms are more frequent where a focal process, such as an atherosclerotic plaque, weakens a portion of the wall allowing it to expand.

MICROSCOPIC FEATURES OF THE AORTA

As many aortic diseases overlap in their microscopic appearance, this section will define microscopic terminology and indicate features to note. To properly diagnose aortic pathology, both H&E and an elastic stain (VVG, Movat, Millers, etc.) are usually needed, although for some histopathologies (inflammatory, neoplastic, purely atherosclerotic) an elastic stain is not entirely necessary. The general construct of the aorta is the lamellar unit which is comprised of a concentric layer of elastic and collagen fibers and the interlamellar zone containing a concentric layer of smooth muscle cells. Injury to the lamellar unit by any of the histopathologies below results in a weakening of the wall and resultant aneurysm.

Inflammation is not a feature of normal aortae and represents a pathologic process. The one exception is the presence of neutrophils palisading around blood vessels in the adventitia, which may represent a response to a long surgery and can be ignored. Inflammatory cell types can vary widely (Fig. 4). Diagnosing an inflammatory process in the aorta, which is often clinically not appreciated, is the key contribution that a pathologist can make on an aortic specimen. The pathologist should be careful to recognize giant cells, eosinophils and plasma cells in addition to a macrophage or lymphocytic infiltrate, as they indicate particular diseases (see below). Generally, adventitial inflammation is lymphocytic/plasmacytic in nature, while medial inflammation is comprised of macrophages and giant cells. Sometimes, this adventitial lymphoplasmacytic inflammation is non-specific to the aortic disease process. If medial inflammation is present, and giant cells are not obviously present, a CD68 stain should be used to improve their recognition.

Medial degeneration (cystic medial degeneration, cystic medial necrosis, cystic medionecrosis, medial necrosis) is denoted by fragmentation and/or loss of elastic fibers in an area of wall degeneration containing a "pool" of glycoprotein (Fig. 5A, B).[6] Medial degeneration is easily appreciated on both H&E and elastic stains (Movat). In the later, the loss of adjacent elastic fibers is apparent.

The histologic appearance of laminar medial necrosis (medionecrosis) is the loss of smooth muscle cells (noted by a lack of their nuclei) in an area of the wall with concomitant elastic fiber collapse. In the absence of elastic fiber collapse, the shorter term 'medial necrosis' is used. This tends to be a patchy process and can be spotted at low power on H&E stained slides in areas where the media is more pink – as a result of fewer basophilic nuclei in the area. On slides stained for elastic fibers, it can be spotted at low power as areas of increased dark staining due to the loss of smooth muscle cells and collapse of the elastic fiber lamellae (see Fig. 5C, D).[6]

Diffuse medial degeneration is a recently described term used to explain the histology of Loeys-Dietz syndrome.[7] It is defined as fragmentation and/or loss of intralamellar elastic fibers with concurrent extracellular matrix deposition (Fig. 6A, B). It does not have the large "pools" of glycoproteins observed in medial degeneration. On an elastic stain, the elastic fibers can be markedly disoriented.

Elastic fiber fragmentation and elastic fiber disorganization are only appreciated on an elastic stain. A normal ascending aorta has regular, thick elastic fibers forming concentric layers from the intima to the adventitia. In this disease process, elastic fibers are notably fragmented, thin, stunted and concurrently lost, such that the overall appearance of the area is significantly paler than normal aorta (see Fig. 6C, D). Remaining fibers can be disorganized, losing their parallel orientation.[2]

Some degree of atherosclerosis is seen in most adult aortae. It can range from a thickened and fibrotic neointima, to a typical atheromatous plaque containing cholesterol clefts, inflammatory cells, calcifications and other features (see Fig. 6E, F). Often the media is thinned below the plaque as a result of chronic ischemia of the vascular smooth muscle cells that are now no longer receiving nutrients directly from the aortic flow.

- At low power, the H&E slide should be evaluated for medial necrosis, medial degeneration, atherosclerosis, and inflammatory infiltrates.
- At medium power, diffuse medial degeneration should be noticeable, although it is often subtle.
- At high power, the types of inflammatory cells, if present, should be noted.
- On an elastic stain, areas of elastic fiber fragmentation and disorientation, laminar medial necrosis, medial degeneration and diffuse medial degeneration can all be noted at medium power.

DIFFERENTIAL DIAGNOSIS AND DIAGNOSIS OF AORTA

Genetic Diseases as Causes of Ascending Aneurysms

In the young adult and pediatric populations, genetic disorders are the predominant cause of

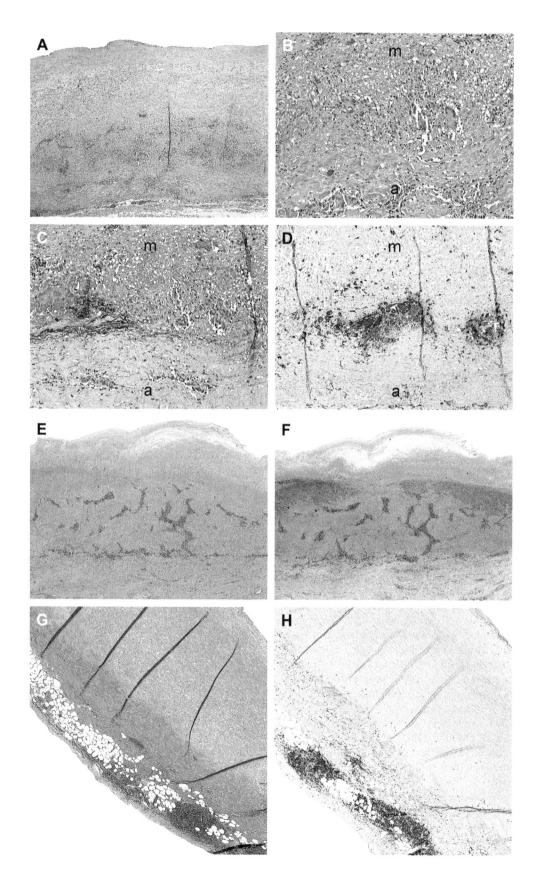

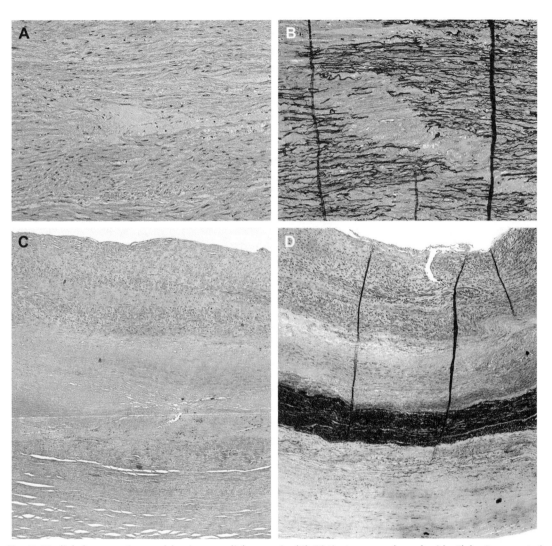

Fig. 5. Medial degeneration and laminar medial necrosis. (*A*) Distinct mucopolysaccharide "lakes" are noted between lamellar units with some localized disorganization of adjacent smooth muscle cells in medial degeneration. (*B*) Elastic fibers are disrupted in areas of medial degeneration. (*C*) At low power medial necrosis can be noted by a general pinkness due to a loss of smooth muscle cell nuclei. (*D*) On a Movat Pentachrome, there is collapse of the elastic fibers into a dense dark band due to the loss of smooth muscle cells.

Fig. 4. Giant cell and lymphoplasmacytic aoritis. (*A*) Low power view of a giant cell inflammation of the aortitis. The inflammation extends predominantly across the outer third of the media and into the adventitia. (*B*) A higher power view shows the destructive inflammatory process containing giant cells along the medial (m) and adventitial (a) junction. (*C*) A Movat Pentachrome shows significant loss of elastic fibers in the media due to the inflammatory process. (*D*) A CD68 IHC stain highlights giant cells. (*E*) Low power view of a lymphoplasmacytic infiltrate predominantly within the medial layer. The intimal and adventitial layers are spared. (*F*) A Movat Pentachrome stain shows a marked loss of elastic fibers in the inflamed region, with residual fibers at the edges of the process. (*G*) A primarily adventitial lymphoplasmacytic infiltrate forming lymphoid aggregates is seen in this specimen. (*H*) A CD3 stain highlights lymphocytes in the adventitia. Longstanding inflammatory processes can cause adventitial thickening.

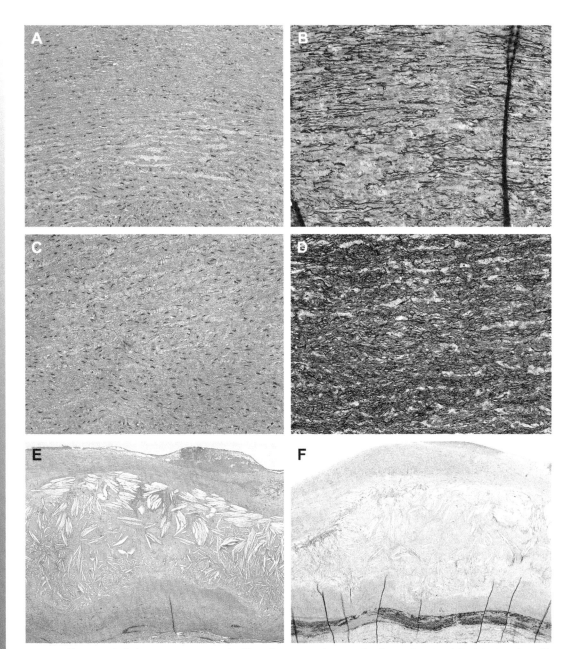

Fig. 6. Diffuse medial degeneration, elastic fiber fragmentation, and atherosclerosis. (*A*) Thin intralamellar collections of pale material are seen in the absence of more extensive "lakes" in diffuse medial degeneration (H&E). (*B*) Often the elastic fibers are disrupted in areas of diffuse medial degeneration and interstitial material becomes more prominent. (*C, D*) On H&E, it is not possible to appreciate the loss and fragmentation of elastic fibers, which are clearly visible on the Movat stain of the same area. (*E, F*) These are the typical findings of a large atheromatous plaque. There is a moderate fibrous cap of neointima overlaying debris including cholesterol clefts. The media is notably thinned with patchy laminar medial necrosis and loss of elastic fibers.

ascending aortic aneurysms and dissections. Most of these disorders have additional physical findings that help clinicians delineate the underlying disease (Table 1).[2] It is not generally possible to make a diagnosis of a specific genetic disease on the histology of the aorta alone. It is therefore a better practice to describe the histologic findings and suggest that they may be the result of a genetic disorder, if that information is not already known. Thus, the specific diagnosis of a genetic

Table 1
Genetic causes of aortic aneurysms

Syndrome	Genetic Mutation	Commonly Associated Systemic Features
Marfan syndrome	FBN1	Arachnodactyly, pectus excavatum, lens ectopia
Vascular Ehlers-Danlos syndrome	COL3A1	Easy bruising, blue/gray sclerae, smooth (velvety) skin
Loeys-Dietz syndrome	TGFBR1, TGFBR2	Bifid or broad uvula, joint laxity, pectus deformities
Turner syndrome	Monosomy X	Webbed neck, lymphedema, poor breast development
Bicuspid aortic valve and aneurysm		None
Arterial tortuosity syndrome	GLUT10	Hernias, cutis laxa, malar hypoplasia
Familial thoracic aortic aneurysm and dissection	MYH11, ACTA2, SMAD3	Hernias, pectus deformities, scoliosis, osteoarthritis (depending on the particular genetic mutation)

Data from Jain D, Dietz HC, Oswald GL, et al. Causes and histopathology of ascending aortic disease in children and young adults. Cardiovasc Pathol 2011;20(1):15–25.

entity based on the aortic specimen is not critical. Following are brief synopses of the most common genetic disorders:

- Marfan Syndrome
- Vascular Ehlers-Danlos Syndrome (vEDS, EDS IV)
- Loeys-Dietz Syndrome
- Turner Syndrome
- Bicuspid Aortic Valve and Aneurysm (BAV)
- Arterial Tortuosity Syndrome
- Familial Thoracic Aortic Aneurysm and Dissection
- Other Rare Genetic Causes of Aortic Aneurysms

MARFAN SYNDROME

Marfan syndrome is classically known for the triad of arachnodactyly (long fingers), pectus excavatum, and lens ectopia. Ascending aneurysms, occurring at the aortic root and including the aortic sinuses occur in 75% of individuals, with some variability based on the particular mutation in the Fibrillin-1 (FBN1) gene.[2] Individuals also have other cardiovascular manifestations including mitral valve prolapse, arrhythmias and cardiomyopathies. Aortae from Marfan syndrome patients frequently have medial degeneration and elastic fiber fragmentation and disorganization.[2,6,8] Laminar medial necrosis is also reported in this population, although it is likely to be encountered more frequently in older individuals.[9] While a mild increase in inflammatory cells has been appreciated around the vasa vasorum, frank inflammation is not a feature of Marfan syndrome.[10] In cases of prophylactic repair, the histologic findings may be subtle or absent – even in genetically proven cases of Marfan syndrome.

VASCULAR EHLERS-DANLOS SYNDROME (vEDS, EDS IV)

This rare and devastating disease is notable for thin skin with visible veins, easy bruising and characteristic facial features. It is caused by mutations in the type 3 procollagen gene (COL3A1), which is an essential collagen in blood vessels and many organs. The mutations cause structural weaknesses and potentially spontaneous ruptures of visceral organs. Although vEDS is grouped with other genetic diseases as causing ascending aortic disease, it causes ruptures at a much higher rate at non-aortic root vascular sites. Many cases of vEDS have no specific histologic pathology making this a difficult diagnostic dilemma.[2] Some cases have reduplication of the internal elastic laminae or evidence of healed small dissections. Electron microscopy can be valuable in these cases where collagen fiber diameter irregularities and extracellular fibrinogranular substance have been reported.[11]

LOEYS-DIETZ SYNDROME

Loeys-Dietz syndrome is a recently described disease with features of both Marfan syndrome and vEDS.[12] Loeys-Dietz syndrome is associated with a bifid uvula, cleft palate, micrognathia, easy bruising and visceral rupture. Loeys-Dietz syndrome is caused by mutations in the transforming growth factor receptors 1 & 2 (*TGFBR1* & *TGFBR2*). This disease has been associated with diffuse medial degeneration and elastic fiber fragmentation and disorganization, rather than medial degeneration, although medial degeneration can rarely be seen in Loeys-Dietz syndrome.[2] The severity of the histologic findings of Loeys-Dietz syndrome associate with the size of aneurysm.[7]

TURNER SYNDROME

Turner syndrome is a disease caused by a complete or partial monosomy of chromosome X (45, X0) and is thus seen exclusively in women. The disease is well-known for the physical features of a webbed-neck, short stature, and lymphedema. Turner syndrome causes a variety of congenital cardiovascular anomalies including aortic aneurysms, elongation of the transverse arch, coarctation, bicuspid aortic valve and partial anomalous pulmonary venous return to the heart. Similar to Marfan syndrome, medial degeneration has been reported as a histopathologic finding in the aortae of Turner syndrome individuals.[9]

BICUSPID AORTIC VALVE AND ANEURYSM (BAV)

Approximately 2% of individuals have a bicuspid aortic valve, making it the most common congenital anomaly of the heart. While many individuals with BAV develop aortic stenosis, a smaller subset develops aortic regurgitation and aneurysm. It appears different genes are involved in these separate outcomes and the gene(s) for aneurysm is currently unknown. This group is susceptible to the same histologic changes–medial degeneration, elastic fiber fragmentation and disorientation, laminar medial necrosis–as seen in other syndromes, although at least one report indicated these changes were less severe than in tricuspid individuals.[2,13]

ARTERIAL TORTUOSITY SYNDROME

This rare disease is notable for runaway vascular growth leading to tortuous vessels throughout the body, dissections and a shortened lifespan. Arterial tortuosity syndrome is caused by mutations in the glucose transporter SLC2A10. Rare histologic reports of this disease indicate elastic fiber fragmentation and concurrent thickened/fibrotic intima.[2]

FAMILIAL THORACIC AORTIC ANEURYSM AND DISSECTION

Approximately 20% of individuals with aortic aneurysms and dissections have a familiar clustering, but do not fit into a particular category described above. A few genes have been described as explaining a small percentage of this population. They are smooth muscle actin, alpha 2 (*ACTA2*), smooth muscle myosin heavy chain 11 (*MYH11*) and *SMAD3*.[14] Medial degeneration and elastic fiber fragmentation and disorganization have been described as histologic findings in this cluster of diseases as well.[2]

OTHER RARE GENETIC CAUSES OF AORTIC ANEURYSMS

Many other diseases are also rarely associated with aortic aneurysms. These diseases include autosomal dominant polycystic kidney disease, Noonan syndrome, tetralogy of Fallot, autosomal recessive cutis laxa, and Sprintzen-Goldberg syndrome. Generally, medial degeneration has been described in rare case reports related to these diseases.[2]

NON GENETIC DISEASE AS A CAUSE OF ASCENDING ANEURYSM

The most common group undergoing ascending aortic aneurysm repair is between ages 59 to 69 years. These individuals are generally thought to have multiple risk factors rather than a Mendelian genetic disease. These risk factors include male sex, age, smoking, hypertension and atherosclerosis. In one report, severe atherosclerotic plaques were found in about 15% of this population.[8] Some of the same histologic features seen in genetic disease are also seen in these older individuals. Laminar medial necrosis is generally believed to be an aging-related process and is seen frequently in this older population (>80%).[8] Elastic fiber fragmentation is frequently present and medial degeneration is routinely reported in these older individuals as well.[15] In this population, a descriptive diagnosis of the aorta, ruling out inflammation and tumor, is generally sufficient.

There are also a few non-genetic diseases that are associated with aortic dissection. Cocaine abuse has been associated with a loss of elasticity, increased aortic stiffness and resultant aortic aneurysm. It can be a significant cause of aortic dissections in inner-city populations.[16] Also, severe physical exertion, particularly weightlifting, is a cause of aortic dissection due to the dramatic elevation of blood pressure in the aorta. For both of these diseases, medial degeneration has been reported, suggesting the potential for underlying subclinical aortic disease.[2]

Inflammatory Diseases

A number of diseases that result in aortic inflammation and aneurysm/dissection have been recognized. Traditionally, a pathologist would attempt to identify a specific clinical disease that related to a histopathologic appearance. That is challenging as it is now understood that there is significant histopathologic and clinical overlap between many diseases and often key clinical characteristics of the patient are unknown to the pathologist. A more recent classification scheme is based purely on the histopathology and simplifies the activity of the pathologist. This section reports on specific known inflammatory entities and concludes with an explanation of the histopathologic-only classification scheme.

- Giant Cell Arteritis
- Takayasu Arteritis
- Syphilitc Aortitis
- Aortitis from IgG4 Related Systemic Disease
- Non-syphilitic Infectious Aortitis

The key concept for the pathologist is to identify the presence of an inflammatory infiltrate and convey this to the clinical team for appropriate follow up. Inflammatory causes of aortic aneurysm are often missed clinically before surgery and they may indicate other systemic diseases or processes that should be treated.

GIANT CELL ARTERITIS

Giant cell arteritis (GCA) can occur in a number of large arterial vessels, most frequently the temporal artery. When GCA affects the aorta it is located in the proximal ascending aorta area. Giant cell aortitis is a complication of a subset of systemic giant cell arteritis cases. If it is confined to the aorta, it can be called "isolated" giant cell aortitis. GCA is, by definition, a disease of the elderly, occurring in individuals older than age 50 years and generally affecting Caucasian women in their 70s. It causes thoracic artery aneurysms in 7% of cases.[17]

Histologically, GCA appears as a granulomatous inflammation of the media, comprised of a polymorphous inflammatory infiltrate of mononuclear histiocytes, lymphocytes, and multinucleated giant cells (see Fig. 4A–D). The inflammation is often patchy and can be missed if tissue sampling is inadequate. In aortic cases with some nonspecific medial macrophage infiltrate, additional sections should be taken of the remaining aortic material to look for giant cells. The granulomatous inflammation is often seen in areas of medial injury. Laminar medial necrosis is a frequent histologic finding in GCA.[3] Giant cells often attack the elastic lamellae at the edges of laminar medial necrosis. Vasa vasorum have been reported to infiltrate deeper into the media in GCA, likely the result of local hypoxia caused by the tissue destruction. The inflammation in GCA is primarily in the media, unlike lymphoplasmacytic aortitis which is more prominent in the adventitia.

TAKAYASU ARTERITIS

Takayasu arteritis is a systemic vasculidity of large vessels than can be present in the aorta. Takayasu arteritis generally involves women less than 40 years of age, although disease in older patients does exist. The incidence of Takayasu arteritis is 100 fold less common than GCA.[17] For individuals between ages 40 to 55 years, where possible overlap with GCA occurs, one should be careful to definitely diagnose either disease. It is good practice to alert the clinician to the histology and recommend it be correlated with the clinical findings, imaging, etc.

Grossly, Takayasu arteritis can have an intimal "tree bark" appearance.[18] Histologically, Takayasu arteritis has an appearance that is similar to GCA with a polymorphous infiltrate comprised of histocytes, lymphocytes, and multinucleated giant cells (see Fig. 4A–D). Some features appear to be more common in Takayasu arteritis relative to GCA. These include a more active and necrotizing inflammatory process containing microabscesses, more giant cells, and more prominent adventitial thickening. However, these histopathologic findings are usually not sufficiently distinct and diagnosis requires differentiation of the diseases on clinical grounds (patient age, additional manifestations, etc).

SYPHILITC AORTITIS

Although syphilis was once a major cause of aortitis, as treatment for syphilis became widely available, this disease entity has become a rare cause of aortitis. However, it is still important that it not be missed. Syphilitic aortitis is caused by the sexually transmitted spirochete *Treponema palladium* and occurs years after initial infection. Syphilitic aortitis occurs exclusively in the ascending aorta with rare extension beyond the descending thoracic aorta.[19]

Grossly, syphilitic aortitis is strongly associated with an intimal "tree bark," which is also seen in Takayasu arteritis.[18] There is gross adventitial thickening, noted histologically by dense fibrous tissue. Most characteristically, the vasa vasora are invariably cuffed by inflammatory cells–predominantly lymphocytes and plasma cells.

This lymphoplasmacytic infiltrate is predominantly in the adventitia, but can extend into the media. The intima and media both have patchy dense fibrous tissue.[20] The media can remain a normal width or can narrow while undergoing elastic fiber fragmentation and laminar medial necrosis concurrent with aneurysmal dilatation. Giant cells can be seen in syphilitic aortitis but are a rare, non-essential feature.[19] Although staining with Warthin-Starry to see spirochetal organisms can be performed, these stains are difficult, if not impossible to interpret due to the similarly staining elastic fibers of the aorta. Rather than performing this staining, serologic testing for syphilis should be recommended to the clinician in cases displaying this histologic picture.[20]

AORTITIS FROM IgG4 RELATED SYSTEMIC DISEASE

In 2001, Hamano discovered that some patients with lymphoplasmacytic sclerosing pancreatitis had high serum levels of IgG4.[21] That began a realization that IgG4 related systemic disease (IgG4-RSD) is the cause of fibroinflammatory processes in multiple organs and vascular sites. It can cause both thoracic and abdominal aortic aneurysms with or without concurrent elevated IgG4 serum levels.[22,23] While most cases of IgG4-RSD aortitis have either been isolated or linked to other fibroinflammatory processes elsewhere in the body, a recent case with IgG4-RSD involving 4 separate blood vessels was described, suggesting the disease may be similar to giant cell arteritis in its ability to involve multiple vessels.[24]

There is only limited information on this entity, although it is likely that some non-specific lymphoplasmacytic aortitis cases of yesteryear, had they been stained for IgG4, would have fit this category. Most individuals have elevated serum IgG4, but it is not required to make this diagnosis. Grossly, the adventitia can be markedly thickened. Histologically, there is a heavy lymphoplasmacytic infiltrate in the adventitia with obstructive phlebitis (**Fig. 7**A, B).[23] In the setting of notable collections of plasma cells, staining should be performed with a CD138 or IgG to determine a baseline level of plasma cells and an IgG4 to determine this specific subpopulation. Although the definitions for the disease are still being debated, the percent of plasma cells that are IgG4 positive should be greater than 50% (see **Fig. 7**C, D).[25] The media can be fairly unremarkable if the infiltrate remains in the adventitia as a periaortitis.[22] In other cases, the infiltrate can appear in the intima and media which can also show elastic fiber fragmentation and laminar medial necrosis.

NON-SYPHILITIC INFECTIOUS AORTITIS

Due to the general resistance of the aorta to infection, infectious aortitis rarely occurs and represents the cause of less than 1% of all aortic repairs.[26] Major risk factors include existing atherosclerotic plaques, immunocompromised patient status, concurrent infectious endocarditis, and aneurysms. Mycotic aneurysms are infected aneurysms which can be the result of secondary infection of an aneurysm or the primary expansion of an aortic wall weakened by infectious aortitis. Gram positive organisms are slightly more common causes of aortitis than gram negative organisms, while fungal causes are exceedingly rare.[27]

Histologically, Miller and colleagues[26] described six patterns that can be seen. The most common was transmural acute (neutrophilic) inflammation with focal microabcesses on a background of calcific intimal atherosclerotic plaques. Another common pattern showed atherosclerosis with marked medial thinning and a chronic inflammatory cell infiltrate. A third pattern included noncaseating granulomatous inflammation of the adventitia and media. The other patterns were rare variants of these three. In general, diffuse neutrophilic or lymphocytic inflammation can be seen in any layer of the blood vessel wall usually in the presence of atherosclerosis. Organismal stains (Gram, etc) should be obtained and can be used to identify bacterial colonies.

HISTOPATHOLOGIC CLASSIFICATION SCHEME OF AORTITIS

In 2008, Drs Burke and Virmani proposed a histologic classification scheme segmenting aortitis into necrotizing and non-necrotizing forms.[28] Necrotizing aortitis was defined by zonal laminar medial necrosis surrounded by giant cells. Non-necrotizing aortitis was characterized by the absence of medial necrosis, but with diffuse medial inflammation of a predominant lymphocytic type. I have found this to be a useful classification scheme, particularly in the absence of clinical information suggesting a specific disease entity.

ABDOMINAL AORTIC ANEURYSMS

Abdominal aortic aneurysms (AAA) is a common disease entity affecting 5 to 7% of men and approximately 1% of women over age 65 years.[29] It is more frequently seen in people with smoking, dyslipidemia and hypertensive risk factors. The

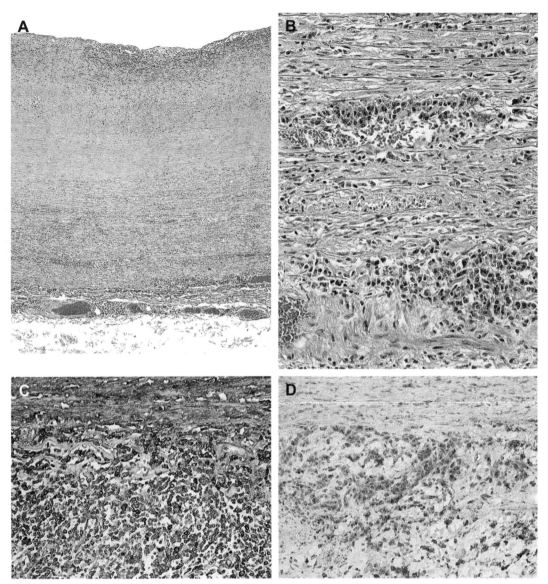

Fig. 7. IgG4 aortitis. (*A*) There is a dense predominantly plasma cell infiltrate that extends from intima into the adventitia. (*B*) At high power, numerous dissecting plasma cells can be seen amongst the medial lamellae. (*C*) An IgG stain is diffusely positive across most of the plasma cells. (*D*) Over 80% of the cells in this view stain positive for IgG4. At least 50% positive staining is recommended to make this diagnosis.

most common histologic finding in these cases is calcific atherosclerosis with resultant thinning of the medial layer. Laminar medial necrosis and elastic fiber fragmentation are invariably present. A small amount of chronic inflammation associated with the atherosclerotic plaque can be present. Where there is more inflammation, than usual, but not enough to clearly be an inflammatory process, this intermediate terminology "atherosclerosis with excessive inflammation"

has been proposed. While most of these specimens are straightforward, one should be aware of excessive inflammation, acute inflammation or granulomatous inflammation as potential signs of infectious aortitis. One should also be aware of marked adventitial thickening as this could represent a fibroinflammatory process. Usually, in this case, the surgeon will have commented on the thickness of the aortic wall, or it's adhesion to other tissues in their surgical report.

UNUSUAL FINDINGS OF SURGICAL AORTAS

- Congenital Abnormalities
- Aortic Tumors
- Fibroinflammatory Disease

Congenital Abnormalities

The primary congenital disease of the aorta is coarctation. This is noted clinically by higher systolic blood pressure in the upper extremities. Coarctations can be congenital or acquired. Coarctation is generally a diagnosis made clinically before surgical repair. Grossly, it is most frequently a narrowing of the aorta distal to the left subclavian artery and before the ligamentum arteriosum, the remnant of the ductus arteriosus. These cases are usually surgically repaired in situ and do not result in intact surgical specimens. However, if a coarctation is removed, the diameter of the aorta before, amidst and beyond the coarctation should be determined. Histologically, the area of coarctation should be evaluated, as the inflammatory process

of Takayasu arteritis and atherosclerosis can both cause aortic narrowing. In congenital cases, medial degeneration is a common.[30] Congenital coarctation is seen in 16% of live Turner syndrome births.[31] Other congenital aortic arch anomalies that may be rarely encountered as surgical specimens are vascular rings and double aortic arches.

Aortic Tumors

The aorta is an extremely rare site for a malignant tumor. Sarcomas are the most frequent primary tumors described although less than 200 are reported in the literature. They are slightly more common among men and occur in the elderly (median age ~60). They generally originate from intimal myofibroblastic cells (Fig. 8A). Grossly they can be large masses that protrude into the aorta and/or cause thinning and aneurysm formation. Histologically, they fall into a variety of well-known sarcoma types. Angiosarcomas, malignant fibrous histiocytomas, leiomyosarcomas, and undifferentiated sarcomas are the most common.

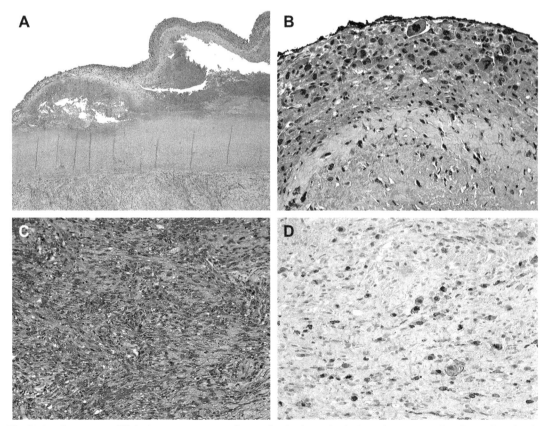

Fig. 8. Aortic sarcoma. (*A*) At low power, tumor is seen both along the intima above necrotic atherosclerotic plaques and within the adventitia below the media. (*B*) At high power, large cells with angulated nuclei and multiple bizarre mitoses are present along the intimal surface. (*C*) Deeper within the tumor, whorls and sheets of mesenchymal appearing cells are present. (*D*) Smooth muscle actin positivity is seen in many tumor cells.

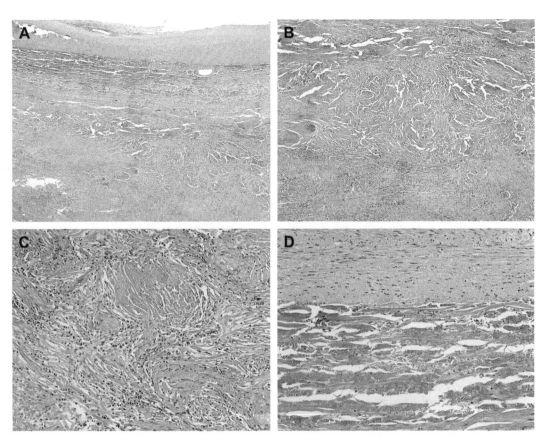

Fig. 9. Fibrosclerosing disease. (*A*) Low power view of the marked adventitial expansion, containing dense collagen, beneath the medial aortic wall. This fibrotic tissue often traps or adheres to other organs. (*B, C*) At higher magnifications, fibroblasts and loose collections of inflammatory cells are appreciated. (*D*) The interface between the media (above) and the adventitia (below) is sharply demarcated.

Histologically, mesenchymal cells, with frequent and bizarre mitoses, expanding the intima are seen (see **Fig. 8**B–D).[32]

Fibroinflammatory Disease

A variety of fibroinflammatory processes are known to occur within the mediastinum and abdomen and involve the aorta. They have been called sclerosing mediastinitis, mediastinal granulomatosis, fibrosing mediastinitis, idiopathic fibroinflammatory lesion of the mediastinum and inflammatory aneurysm of the aorta.[33] All of these entities are generally a fibrotic process of unknown etiology that begins in the mediastinum or abdomen and can trap, compress or infiltrate the aorta or other vessels and nerves.[34] Often there are dense adhesions of the adventitial surface of the aorta to other organs or structures, making the surgical resection challenging. Grossly these masses have a range of appearances: tan-yellow to gray-white and gelatinous to firm. Histologically,

these cases have been classified into three grades. They range from myxomatous connective tissue with abundant spindle cells to dense hyalinized collagen in strands and whorls with few to no spindle-cells (**Fig. 9**). Chronic inflammatory cells, predominantly lymphocytes, plasma cells and macrophages are typically present as well

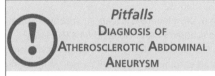

Pitfalls
DIAGNOSIS OF
ATHEROSCLEROTIC ABDOMINAL
ANEURYSM

! Acute inflammation, extensive chronic inflammation and granulomas may be the result of an infectious aortitis

! Thickened adventitia may be the result of a fibroinflammatory disease at all grades. Necrosis and granulomatous in-flammation are not features of this process.

REFERENCES

1. Stone JR, Basso C, Baandrup UT, et al. Recommendations for processing cardiovascular surgical pathology specimens: a consensus statement from the Standards and Definitions Committee of the Society for Cardiovascular Pathology and the Association for European Cardiovascular Pathology. Cardiovasc Pathol 2012;21(1):2–16.

2. Jain D, Dietz HC, Oswald GL, et al. Causes and histopathology of ascending aortic disease in children and young adults. Cardiovasc Pathol 2011; 20(1):15–25.

3. Miller DV, Maleszewski JJ. The pathology of large-vessel vasculitides. Clin Exp Rheumatol 2011;29(1 Suppl 64):S92–8.

4. Gravanis MB. Giant cell arteritis and Takayasu aortitis: morphologic, pathogenetic and etiologic factors. Int J Cardiol 2000;75(Suppl 1):S21–33 [discussion: S35–6].

5. van Dijk RA, Virmani R, von der Thusen JH, et al. The natural history of aortic atherosclerosis: a systematic histopathological evaluation of the peri-renal region. Atherosclerosis 2010;210(1):100–6.

6. Homme JL, Aubry MC, Edwards WD, et al. Surgical pathology of the ascending aorta: a clinicopathologic study of 513 cases. Am J Surg Pathol 2006;30(9): 1159–68.

7. Maleszewski JJ, Miller DV, Lu J, et al. Histopathologic findings in ascending aortas from individuals with Loeys-Dietz syndrome (LDS). Am J Surg Pathol 2009;33(2):194–201.

8. Nesi G, Anichini C, Tozzini S, et al. Pathology of the thoracic aorta: a morphologic review of 338 surgical specimens over a 7-year period. Cardiovasc Pathol 2009;18(3):134–9.

9. Halushka MK. Single gene disorders of the aortic wall. Cardiovasc Pathol 2012. [Epub ahead of print].

10. Guo G, Booms P, Halushka M, et al. Induction of macrophage chemotaxis by aortic extracts of the mgR Marfan mouse model and a GxxPG-containing fibrillin-1 fragment. Circulation 2006; 114(17):1855–62.

11. Germain DP, Herrera-Guzman Y. Vascular Ehlers-Danlos syndrome. Ann Genet 2004;47(1):1–9.

12. Loeys BL, Chen J, Neptune ER, et al. A syndrome of altered cardiovascular, craniofacial, neurocognitive and skeletal development caused by mutations in TGFBR1 or TGFBR2. Nat Genet 2005; 37(3):275–81.

13. Matthias Bechtel JF, Noack F, Sayk F, et al. Histopathological grading of ascending aortic aneurysm: comparison of patients with bicuspid versus tricuspid aortic valve. J Heart Valve Dis 2003;12(1):54–9 [discussion: 59–61].

14. van de Laar IM, Oldenburg RA, Pals G, et al. Mutations in SMAD3 cause a syndromic form of aortic aneurysms and dissections with early-onset osteoarthritis. Nat Genet 2011;43(2):121–6.

15. Brinster DR, Rizzo RJ, Bolman RM. Ascending aortic aneurysms. In: Cohn LH, editor. Cardiac surgery in the adult. New York: McGraw Hill; 2007. p. 1223–49.

16. Hsue PY, Salinas CL, Bolger AF, et al. Acute aortic dissection related to crack cocaine. Circulation 2002;105(13):1592–5.

17. Richards BL, March L, Gabriel SE. Epidemiology of large-vessel vasculidities. Best Pract Res Clin Rheumatol 2010;24(6):871–83.

18. Tavora F, Burke A. Review of isolated ascending aortitis: differential diagnosis, including syphilitic, Takayasu's and giant cell aortitis. Pathology 2006; 38(4):302–8.

19. Heggtveit HA. Syphilitic Aortitis. A clinicopathologic autopsy study of 100 cases, 1950 to 1960. Circulation 1964;29:346–55.

20. Roberts WC, Ko JM, Vowels TJ. Natural history of syphilitic aortitis. Am J Cardiol 2009;104(11):1578–87.

21. Hamano H, Kawa S, Horiuchi A, et al. High serum IgG4 concentrations in patients with sclerosing pancreatitis. N Engl J Med 2001;344(10):732–8.

22. Kasashima S, Zen Y. IgG4-related inflammatory abdominal aortic aneurysm. Curr Opin Rheumatol 2011;23(1):18–23.

23. Stone JR. Aortitis, periaortitis, and retroperitoneal fibrosis, as manifestations of IgG4-related systemic disease. Curr Opin Rheumatol 2011;23(1):88–94.

24. Holmes BJ, Delev NG, Pasternack GR, et al. Vascular survey in IgG4-related systemic disease. Mod Pathol 2012;25(Suppl 2):79A.

25. Stone JH, Zen Y, Deshpande V. IgG4-related disease. N Engl J Med 2012;366(6):539–51.

26. Miller DV, Oderich GS, Aubry MC, et al. Surgical pathology of infected aneurysms of the descending thoracic and abdominal aorta: clinicopathologic correlations in 29 cases (1976 to 1999). Hum Pathol 2004;35(9):1112–20.

27. Lopes RJ, Almeida J, Dias PJ, et al. Infectious thoracic aortitis: a literature review. Clin Cardiol 2009;32(9):488–90.

28. Burke AP, Tavora F, Narula N, et al. Aortitis and ascending aortic aneurysm: description of 52 cases and proposal of a histologic classification. Hum Pathol 2008;39(4):514–26.

29. Krishna SM, Dear AE, Norman PE, et al. Genetic and epigenetic mechanisms and their possible role in abdominal aortic aneurysm. Atherosclerosis 2010; 212(1):16–29.

30. Isner JM, Donaldson RF, Fulton D, et al. Cystic medial necrosis in coarctation of the aorta: a potential factor contributing to adverse

consequences observed after percutaneous balloon angioplasty of coarctation sites. Circulation 1987;75(4):689–95.

31. Kim HK, Gottliebson W, Hor K, et al. Cardiovascular anomalies in Turner syndrome: spectrum, prevalence, and cardiac MRI findings in a pediatric and young adult population. AJR Am J Roentgenol 2011;196(2):454–60.

32. Chiche L, Mongredien B, Brocheriou I, et al. Primary tumors of the thoracoabdominal aorta: surgical treatment of 5 patients and review of the literature. Ann Vasc Surg 2003;17(4):354–64.

33. Jain D, Fishman EK, Argani P, et al. Unexpected sclerosing mediastinitis involving the ascending aorta in the setting of a multifocal fibrosclerotic disorder. Pathol Res Pract 2011;207(1):60–2.

34. Flieder DB, Suster S, Moran CA. Idiopathic fibroinflammatory (fibrosing/sclerosing) lesions of the mediastinum: a study of 30 cases with emphasis on morphologic heterogeneity. Mod Pathol 1999;12(3):257–64.

SURGICAL PATHOLOGY OF SMALL- AND MEDIUM-SIZED VESSELS

Michael A. Seidman, MD, PhD,
Richard N. Mitchell, MD, PhD*

KEYWORDS

- Artery • Arteriole • Capillary • Vein • Venule • Blood vessel • Aneurysm • Arteritis • Vasculitis
- Atherosclerosis • Thrombosis • Embolism

ABSTRACT

Surgical pathologists encounter blood vessels in virtually every specimen they receive, but pathologies intrinsic to the vessels themselves are distinctly less common. Nevertheless, there are a variety of specific diagnoses and procedures involving vascular specimens that merit the attention of the anatomic pathologist. Etiologically, such pathologies can be broadly grouped into traumatic, degenerative, congenital, inflammatory, infectious, and neoplastic lesions. Major examples of most of these are discussed, including anuerysms, vasculitis, thrombosis/embolism, and atherosclerosis.

GENERAL PATHOLOGIC CONSIDERATIONS FOR VESSELS

Surgical specimens removed for vascular pathology include the vessels themselves, usually medium-to-large sized arteries or veins, as well as vessel contents. Additionally, vascular disease may involve viscera, and as such some of the findings described in this article occur in biopsies or larger tissue resections. The pathologies, both for primary vascular specimens and vascular diseases within viscera, fall into a number of broad categories.

A large portion of vessel pathology results from acquired damage, either in the form of acute trauma or chronic degeneration. Weakened vessel walls of any etiology can result in aneurysm, dissection, or rupture. The major role of the surgical pathologist in examining such specimens is to either confirm clinical suspicions or to suggest underlying etiologies, recognition of which may influence therapy (eg, in the case of infection or primary vasculitis).

Congenital lesions involving the vessels are commonly attributable to defects in extracellular matrix or smooth muscle organization and manifest as aneurysms, dissections, or arterio-venous malformations. While frequently involving the aorta (see the article by Halushka elsewhere in this issue), smaller branches – arteries and arterioles – can also be affected.

Inflammatory disease, ie, vasculitis, can involve any blood vessel; some of the most common primary vasculitides are addressed below. It is important to note that not all inflammation surrounding a blood vessel is necessarily vasculitis; rather, the terminology should be limited to primary inflammatory pathologies and should exclude lesions where vessels are secondarily inflamed in the context of broader inflammation.

Vessels can be involved by disease spread from other sites in the body; thus infections can involve vessel walls and present as aneurysms and/or vasculitis. Emboli should also be examined histologically to establish whether these are primarily thrombotic, infectious, or neoplastic in origin.

ANEURYSMAL DISEASE

Aneurysms of medium-sized arteries occur in a number of contexts (for aortic aneurysms, see

Department of Pathology, Brigham & Women's Hospital/Harvard Medical School, 75 Francis Street, Boston, MA 02115, USA
* Corresponding author.
E-mail address: rmitchell@rics.bwh.harvard.edu

the article by Halushka elsewhere in this issue). The common etiologies include "degenerative" (eg, secondary to hypertension or atherosclerosis), congenital, or infectious.

GROSS ASSESSMENT

Aneurysmal vessel resections should be grossly evaluated for wall thickening, thinning, calcification (distinguishing between intimal and medial calcification), and dissection or rupture. The diameter of the uninvolved and involved segments should be recorded separately. After fixation and, if required, decalcification, the specimen should be sectioned longitudinally to sample the shoulder of the aneurysm, including both normal and pathologic vessel wall in one section. This allows for histologic comparison of the architecture between the two segments.

MICROSCOPIC FEATURES

Microscopic evaluation involves an assessment of all three layers of the vessel wall: intima, media, and adventitia.

Intimal thickness, degree of lipid/cholesterol deposition, inflammatory infiltrate, degree of smooth muscle proliferation, and presence or absence of thrombus on the endothelial surface are all important considerations.

Medial evaluation includes assessment of thickness, presence of inflammatory infiltrate, degenerative changes (eg, diminished smooth muscle content or increased myxomatous matrix), and presence of calcification.

Adventitial changes may include fibrosis and/or chronic inflammation. Care should be taken to distinguish hemorrhage or trauma caused by the

surgical procedure versus lesions present before surgical excision.

PATTERN RECOGNITION

Congenital syndromes that predispose to aneurysm fall under the broader category of diseases known as fibromuscular dysplasia (FMD).[1,2] The primary finding is focally attenuated and even occasionally absent media with fibrous replacement (Fig. 1). Such medial drop-out with or without an aneurysm suggests the diagnosis of FMD. Trichrome or elastic stains may be helpful in evaluating the findings of FMD, but no definite histologic criteria for diagnosing FMD have been published. Specific etiologies for FMD include Ehler-Danlos Syndrome (EDS) Type IV and neurofibromatosis (NF) Type I; confirmation of these diagnoses requires genetic testing.[3] Family history in such cases can be variable, as some of the conditions are recessively inherited, are variably penetrant, and/or can develop de novo.

Aneurysms secondary to infection ("mycotic" aneurysms) will typically show prominent neutrophilic infiltrates, often with hemorrhage and/or tissue necrosis; in the absence of prior antibiotic therapy, microorganisms should be evident on special stains (eg, Gram, methenamine silver, etc; Fig. 2). The most commonly identified organisms in such cases are Gram-positive cocci from oral or skin sources.[4]

In the absence of findings suggesting congenital or infectious etiology, evaluation should focus on recognition of acquired degenerative changes. Atherosclerotic plaque, with intimal thickening, chronic inflammation, and lipid rich cores, can be associated with medial remodeling or necrosis due to inflammatory mediators, matrix metalloproteinase elaboration, and ischemia due to the thickened intima and increased diffusion distance. If severe, these changes can induce substantial medial attenuation. This secondary loss of medial integrity in the context of a friable intima is often associated with aneurysmal dilation, particularly in larger aortic branches, eg, the carotid and renal arteries.

Hypertensive changes include intimal hyperplasia and medial hypertrophy, particularly evident in the vessels of the vasa vasorum. Medial degeneration, while not specific for hypertensive damage, manifests as loss of medial smooth muscle nuclei with increased myxoid extracellular matrix accumulation.

Aneurysms can also be secondary to inflammatory degeneration; in such cases, findings of an occult arteritis may be seen (see below).

Microvascular disease secondary to diabetes or chronic renal disease can occasionally be

Key Considerations
ANEURYSMAL DISEASE

1. The surgical pathologist's primary role in aneurysmal disease is to suggest possible etiologies that may have implications for future therapy and/or familial screening.

2. Aneurysmal vessel resection specimens should be evaluated grossly and microscopically with longitudinal sections to assess features in all three vessel wall layers in both normal and pathologic regions of the specimen.

3. Etiologies include congenital, infectious, degenerative, and inflammatory.

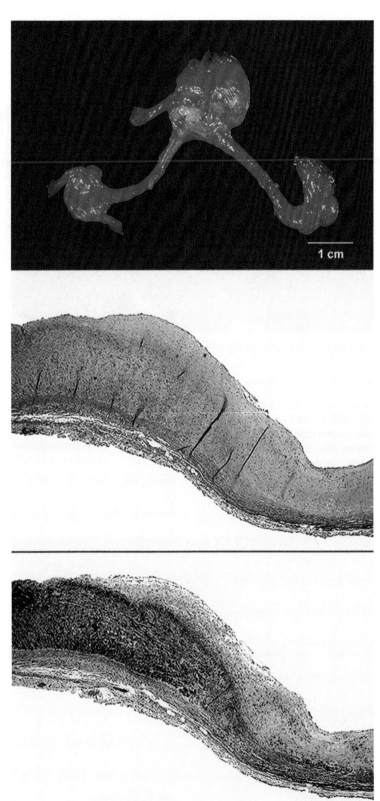

Fig. 1. Fibromuscular dysplasia. This splenic artery segment, involved by several aneurysms (*upper panel*), showed loss of the media with intimal fibrosis in the areas of aneurysm (*middle* and *lower panels*, aneurysm on the right side of the field). Middle panel: H&E stain. Lower panel: Modified Masson trichrome stain.

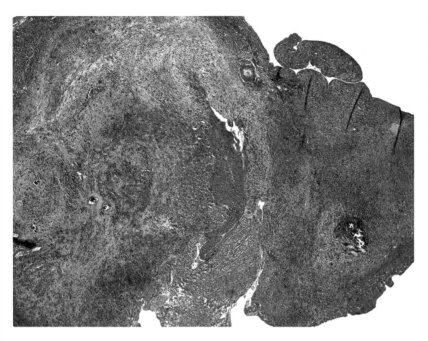

Fig. 2. Mycotic aneurysm. The wall of this vessel, sampled from an area of cerebral aneurysm, shows significant damage with acute and chronic inflammation, with hemorrhage and fibrin deposition. Special stains and clinical cultures revealed bacteria present within the tissue.

suggested by intimal hyperplasia (not necessarily associated with calcification or atherosclerosis) and medial calcification (ie, Mönckeberg's calcification, **Fig. 3**), the latter most commonly at the medial aspect of the internal elastic lamina.

PROGNOSIS/FAMILIAL RISK

Once identified, repair (endovascular or surgical) is generally successful for managing medium-vessel aneurysms. The pathologist is important

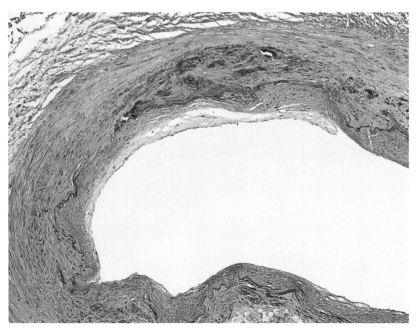

Fig. 3. Mönckeberg's calcification. Calcification in the media of a vessel, often in close proximity to the internal elastic lamina, as shown here, is classified as Mönckeberg's calcification, a distinct entity from atherosclerosis. This pattern of calcification is commonly associated with metabolic dysregulation such as that seen in renal failure.

Pitfalls
ANEURYSMAL DISEASE

! Medial attenuation may be secondary to acquired degenerative changes and does not automatically indicate a congenital or inflammatory etiology.

! Failure to recognize possible congenital or inflammatory etiologies can have significant clinical consequences.

! Transverse sections may not reveal congenital lesions such as fibromuscular dysplasia.

for identifying potential underlying conditions (including systemic etiologies) that may require specific therapy. Additionally, identification of a congenital etiology (ie, FMD) carries potential screening implications for family members.

ARTERITIS

Inflammation of arteries, ie, arteritis, is a collection of diseases characterized by active inflammation within the media of the arterial wall. The most common vasculitis specimen encountered by a surgical pathologist is the temporal artery biopsy, submitted for assessment of giant cell arteritis (GCA), also known as temporal arteritis. This disease is spatially and temporally heterogeneous throughout the entire carotid tree and aortic arch, with rare cases showing comparable pathology in the subdiaphragmatic aorta.

Key Considerations
GIANT CELL ARTERITIS

1. Proper processing of the gross specimen is essential to proper interpretation of the biopsy.

2. A minimum post-fixation length of 1.0 cm is currently recommended for an adequate temporal artery biopsy.

3. The diagnosis of active arteritis requires documentation of inflammation in the media.

4. The diagnosis of healed arteritis requires contiguous loss of at least 20% of the internal elastic lamina, medial attenuation and/or neovascularization, and adventitial fibrosis.

GROSS ASSESSMENT/TISSUE PROCESSING

The temporal artery is biopsied because it is superficial and therefore easy to access, and because circulation in the area is redundant and the vessel can be safely sacrificed. To assess for GCA, the longer the biopsy the better, in light of the patchy nature of the pathology; current recommendations typically suggest a biopsy length of at least 1.0 cm.[5,6]

The length of the segment should be noted as a measure of specimen adequacy; width should also be recorded, but is less useful in diagnosis. Blood, muscle, adipose, and other non-vascular tissues should be noted to aid in microscopic assessment and in clinical correlation of side-effects from surgery. The specimen should be submitted entirely in one piece to the histology laboratory, with specific instructions:

- After tissue processing, the specimen should be cut by the embedding technician approximately every 0.3 cm along the vessel length and all sections should be embedded in cross section.
- Three (3) adjacent tissue profiles should be cut on each of five (5) levels/slides.
- The first, third, and fifth slide should be stained with H&E, and the second and fourth slides should be stained with an elastic stain.

In processing other biopsy specimens for arteritis, similar procedures should be implemented; arteritis should always be evaluated on a cross section of the vessel.

MICROSCOPIC FEATURES

GCA is characterized by a predominantly lymphohistiocytic infiltrate in the vessel media (a finding required to diagnose active arteritis), most commonly centered on the internal elastic lamina (IEL; **Fig. 4**). Inflammation may extend to the intima and/or adventitia, including formation of lymphoid follicles in the adventitia, but these findings are neither required nor specific. Although assiduous examination and multiple levels will usually expose at least one multinucleated giant cell, these need not be present and are not seen in some 20 to 30% of GCA patients. Intimal disruption or hyperplasia may also be seen. Disruption of the IEL is seen with established disease, and usually involves more than a contiguous quarter of the diameter with underlying medial attenuation, neovascularization, and/or adventitial fibrosis. Luminal stenosis and/or thrombosis can also occur.

In the absence of medial inflammation, the findings of at least 20% continuous circumferential

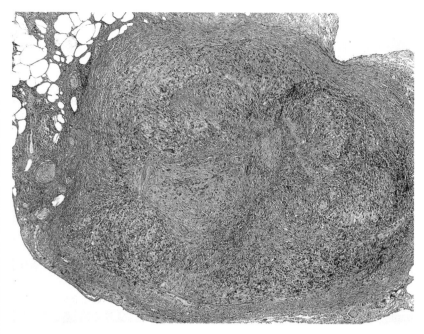

Fig. 4. Temporal artery biopsy, active giant cell arteritis (GCA). During the active phase of GCA, chronic inflammation is identified in the media of the vessel. While not required for the diagnosis, there may be extensive inflammation with formation of giant cells and granulomas, focal fibrinoid necrosis of the vessel wall, luminal obliteration, significant destruction of the internal elastic lamina, and adventitial fibrosis. H&E stain.

disruption of the IEL, medial attenuation and/or neovascularization, and adventitial fibrosis together make up the constellation of findings currently diagnosed as "healed arteritis" (**Fig. 5**).[7,8] This diagnosis is most consistent with prior arteritis at the site of the biopsy but with no activity at the site currently; the disease may be concurrently active at other vascular sites, including immediately adjacent vessel segments. The same findings may be seen in "burned out" arteritis of any type.

Intimal hyperplasia and elastic tissue reduplication can be secondary to a large number of diseases, including atherosclerosis, hypertension, diabetic vasculopathy, trauma, or arteritis; these findings are therefore non-specific (**Fig. 6**). Trauma and aging may also be associated with focal disruption of the IEL (typically <20% of the circumference), as can Mönckeberg's calcification, a metabolic medial calcification commonly seen in patients with renal insufficiency. Mild adventitial fibrosis itself is also a non-specific finding. Given current data, only the full constellation of findings described above (extensive elastic tissue fragmentation, medial attenuation and/or neovascularization, and adventitial fibrosis) can be attributed to remote vasculitis in the absence of concurrent, active medial inflammation.

PROGNOSIS

GCA can be managed with corticosteroids with a good prognosis. Untreated, the condition can lead to blindness, via involvement of the retinal artery, or subarachnoid hemorrhage, via involvement of the intracranial arteries. The prognosis for patients that show only the residua of prior inflammation appears likewise favorable, although there are no definitive treatment recommendations for a diagnosis of "healed arteritis."

Pitfalls
GIANT CELL ARTERITIS

! Do not haphazardly embed temporal artery biopsies – proper handling is mandatory.

! Giant cells are not required to diagnose giant cell arteritis.

! Do not confuse degenerative changes, eg, intimal thickening and elastic tissue reduplication, with healed arteritis.

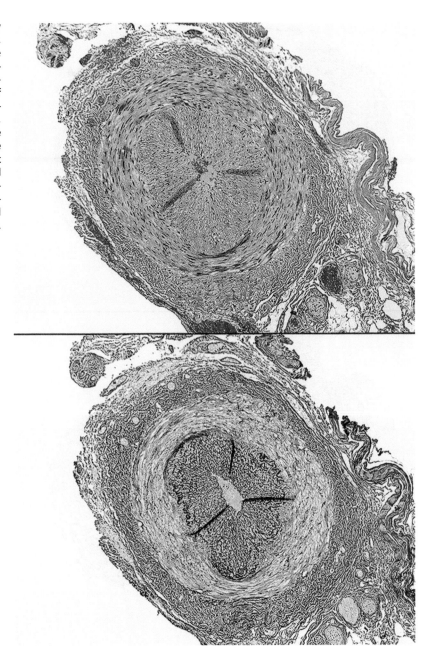

Fig. 5. Temporal artery biopsy, healed arteritis. With resolution of the active inflammatory component of giant cell arteritis, several sequelae of the disease can be identified that, in combination, are relatively suggestive of the diagnosis. These include destruction of at least 20% of the internal elastic lamina, medial attenuation and/or neovascularization, and adventitial fibrosis. Upper: H&E stain. Lower: Elastic stain.

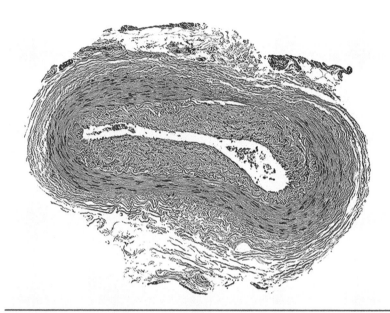

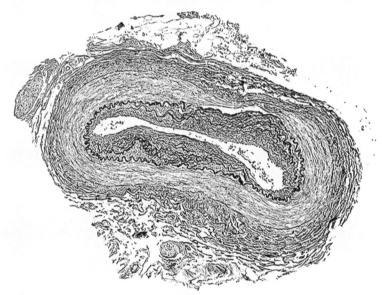

Fig. 6. Temporal artery biopsy, negative for vasculitis. Normal aging, particularly in the context of chronic hypertension or prior trauma, can cause changes to the temporal artery to include intimal hyperplasia, focal damage to the internal elastic lamina, elastic tissue reduplication, focal medial attenuation, and mild adventitial fibrosis. Upper: H&E stain. Lower: Elastic stain.

SMALL VESSEL VASCULITIS

Small vessel vasculitis has a variety of etiologies and clinical manifestations.[9] Some are associated with anti-neutrophil cytoplasmic antibodies (ANCA) directed against neutrophil intracellular antigens, including Churg-Strauss syndrome (also called allergic angiitis) and Wegener's granulomatosis (now known as granulomatosis with polyangiitis, GPA). Polyarteritis nodosa (PAN) exists in variants with and without associated ANCA. Leukocytoclastic vasculitis is a family of small vessel vasculitides

Key Considerations
SMALL VESSEL VASCULITIS

1. Vasculitides are classified by the size of the vessel involved, the anatomic sites involved, and the nature of the inflammatory infiltrate.

2. Clinical correlation is essential for properly classifying many forms of small vessel vasculitis.

associated with immune complex deposition, most commonly seen in the skin in association with palpable purpura. Buerger's disease (thromboangiitis obliterans) is a disease of inflammatory/thrombotic occlusion of medium- and small-sized arteries etiologically associated with smoking. Behçet's disease is a neutrophilic vasculitis classically involving the oral and genital mucosa, and other sites.

GROSS ASSESSMENT

Vasculitides are most commonly diagnosed on biopsies or resections of skin, mucosa, or viscera;

the specimen should be processed as appropriate for the type of biopsy. Gross evaluation may suggest an inflammatory process or necrotizing lesion, but the diagnosis is primarily microscopic.

MICROSCOPIC FEATURES

As noted previously, a diagnosis of vasculitis involving arteries (arteritis) requires inflammation involving the media. It is important to evaluate vessels away from areas of large tissue destruction; vascular inflammatory infiltrates there are a more reliable indicator of vasculitis. Conversely,

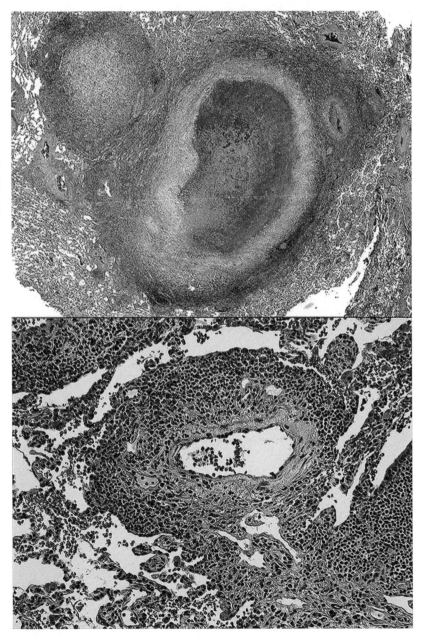

Fig. 7. Wegener's granulomatosis/Granulomatosis with polyangiitis (GPA). This lung section shows well formed granulomas with so-called "dirty" necrosis and a well defined border showing an organized lymphohistiocytic inflammation (*upper panel*, H&E stain). Outside of these granulomas, arteries can be identified that show extensive medial inflammation, including some eosinophils (*lower panel* H&E stain).

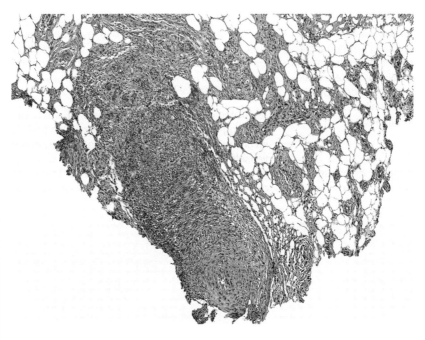

Fig. 8. Polyarteritis nodosa (PAN). This subcutaneous arteriole shows extensive inflammatory infiltrate in the media. Such medium-sized vessel vasculitis in the appropriate clinical context is consistent with a diagnosis of PAN. H&E stain.

secondary involvement of vessels, eg, in areas of necrosis, can mimic vasculitis but should not be used for diagnosis. Inflammation of the intima (endotheliitis) can be a manifestation of vasculitis, but should be categorized separately since it may reflect only superficial endothelial activation and/or intravascular leukocyte activation. Inflammation involving the adventitia around a vessel in isolation can be non-specific and is not sufficient for a vasculitis diagnosis. Elastic stains demonstrating internal elastic lamina disruption may occasionally be helpful.

In ANCA-associated vasculitis, the inflammation is typically mixed with lymphocytes, histiocytes, eosinophils, and neutrophils; damage secondary to the destruction of vessels can create mucosal

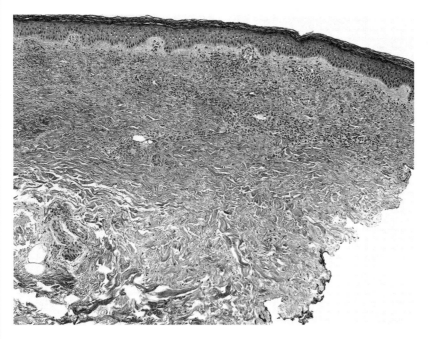

Fig. 9. Leukocytoclastic vasculitis (LCV). Inflammation of the wall of small vessels, such as the dermal arterioles and capillaries shown in this image, is classified as LCV. H&E stain.

Fig. 10. Thromboangiitis obliterans. Arteritis with associated thrombosis and luminal obliteration is the histologic hallmark of thromboangiitis obliterans, also known as Buerger's disease, most commonly seen in young male smokers. In chronic cases, recanalization of the lumen may begin, with possible involvement of those neovessels in the inflammatory process. H&E stain.

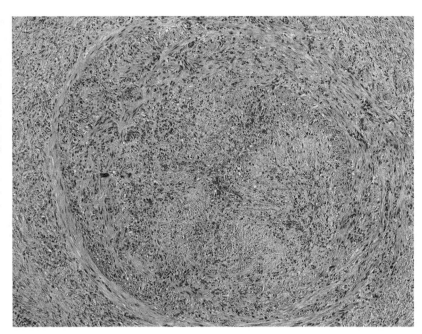

ulceration (eg, in the nasal sinuses) or mass lesions (eg, in the lung). Churg-Strauss is classically associated with eosinophilic infiltrates. Wegener's/GPA can have scattered eosinophils, but is better characterized by a granulomatous inflammation (**Fig. 7**). PAN, both in the ANCA-associated and classic forms, is a mixed inflammation, although more commonly involving smaller vessels and much less

commonly containing eosinophils (**Fig. 8**). The distinction between these three is best made based on site of involvement and clinical consideration.

Leukocytoclastic vasculitis, including Henoch-Schönlein Purpura (HSP) and cryoglobulinemic vasculitis, is restricted to small vessels, most commonly post-capillary venules, and can show any mix of inflammatory cells (**Fig. 9**). Neutrophils

Fig. 11. Behçet's disease. Lesions caused by Behcet's show a neutrophilic inflammation involving the small vessels in the absence of any infectious agent. Shown is a tongue biopsy from a patient with clinically-confirmed disease. H&E stain.

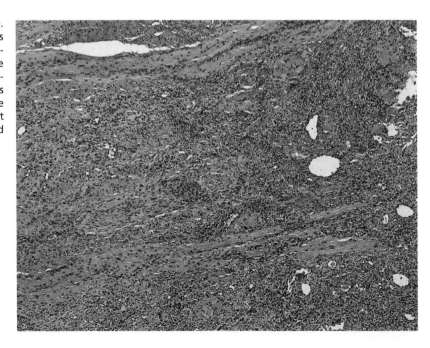

typically predominate in early lesions but diminish as lesions evolve. Deposition of immunoglobulin subtypes or complement proteins (as demonstrated by immunofluorescence) will help solidify a diagnosis.

Buerger's disease is characterized by transmural inflammation, most often neutrophilic, with associated thrombus formation (Fig. 10). The disease is classified by a set of clinical criteria including involvement of extremities and a history of smoking. The role of the pathologist is to exclude other vasculitides, trauma, or infection as alternate etiologies.

Behçet's disease is characterized by dense vessel wall neutrophilic infiltrates (Fig. 11). Again, the diagnosis requires clinical correlation (eg,

Table 1
Features of common vasculitides

	Giant Cell Arteritis (GCA)	Wegener's Granulomatosis/ Granulomatosis with Polyangiitis (GPA)	Churg-Strauss Syndrome (CSS)	Polyarteritis Nodosa (PAN)	Leukocytoclastic Vasculitis (LCV)	Buerger's Disease	Behçet's Disease
Sites of involvement							
Aorta	+	−	−	−	−	−	−
Medium-sized arteries	+	+	+	+	−	+	+
Small-sized arteries	−	+	+	+	+	+	+
Capillaries	−	−	−	−	+	−	+
Veins	−	−	−	−	+	+	+
Central nervous system	−	+	+	+	+	−	+
Eyes	+	+	−	−	−	−	+
Gastrointestinal	−	−	+	+	+	−	+
Heart	−	−	+	+	+	−	rare
Inner ear	−	+	−	−	−	−	+
Joints	−	+	+	+	+	−	+
Kidney	−	+	+	+	+	−	−
Lung	−	+	+	+	+	−	+
Muscles	−	−	+	+	+	−	+
Nerves	−	+	+	+	+	−	+
Skin	−	+	+	+	+	−	+
Upper Airway	−	+	−	−	−	−	−
Inflammatory cells present							
Lymphocytes	+	+	+	±	±	±	±
Histiocytes	+	+	+	±	±	±	±
Neutrophils	rare	+	+	±	±	±	required
Eosinophils	very rare	±	required	±	±	±	±
Other features							
Granulomas	±[a]	required[a]	±	−	−	−	−
Giant cells	often; not required	±	−	−	−	−	−
Thrombosis	±	±	±	±	±	required	±
Serum ANCA positivity	−	+	+	±	−	−	−
Clinical history	>40 y.o., ± polymyalgia rheumatica (PMR)	any	asthma, atopy	any	any	young male smoker	orogenital ulcers

±, Indicates that the finding may or may not be present.
[a] The granulomas of GCA are found within the vessel wall as part of the inflammation comprising the vasculitis, but need not be present to render the diagnosis. The granulomas of GPA are larger, spanning between vessels, and associated with areas of tissue necrosis.

mucosal ulceration) and no specific histologic criteria exist.

The various vasculitides are summarized in **Table 1**.

PROGNOSIS

Most of the vasculitides respond well to immunosuppressive therapy and/or withdrawal of antigenic stimuli (eg, smoking cessation) and can be managed long-term with a favorable prognosis.

ATHEROSCLEROSIS

Atherosclerosis is extremely common, and should always be considered when evaluating arterial specimens. It is most commonly encountered in medium- and large-sized vessels, can vary in severity within different sites within the same patient, and may be calcified, hemorrhagic, or exhibit dense inflammation.[10] While recognition of the diagnosis is typically sufficient, characterization of more subtle features may be germane as we learn more about this condition.

GROSS ASSESSMENT

No special processing is required to evaluate atherosclerosis per se; sections should demonstrate the vessel wall in cross section from intima to adventitia to assess the extent of luminal stenosis. Gross assessment of the apparent magnitude of disease

Key Considerations
ATHEROSCLEROSIS

1. Atherosclerosis is characterized by intimal hyperplasia, chronic inflammation, and lipid accumulation.

2. Mönckeberg's calcification is a distinct medial process associated with renal disease and other metabolic dysregulation.

3. Evidence of prior thrombosis and/or attenuation of cap fibrosis can suggest plaque instability.

(eg, mild, moderate, or severe) and degree of occlusion, the presence or absence of calcification, and the relative thickness of any appreciable fibrous cap on the plaques is important although better assessed histologically. Vessels should be decalcified before cutting serial sections; multiple cross sections can be submitted in the same cassette.

MICROSCOPIC FEATURES

Histologically, atherosclerosis is characterized by scattered mononuclear inflammatory cells (mostly macrophages) with lipid accumulation, typically appearing as cholesterol clefts and foam cells (**Fig. 12**). Intimal-based smooth muscle proliferation is a cardinal feature of the disease. Calcification within atherosclerotic plaque is important to distinguish from medial calcification (Mönckeberg's). The intimal aspect of the plaque will typically have a fibrous cap, and the relative thickness of this cap should be noted to aid in distinguishing stable plaques (those likely to continue to stenose slowly without rupture) from unstable plaques (those likely to rupture and thrombose suddenly).

It is important to examine the endothelial surface for evidence of mural thrombus, as this is indicative of plaque rupture or erosion, and can be suggestive of past or potential future infarction events. Organized thrombus suggests a more remote event, and can help judge chronicity. Recanalization of plaques with small capillaries also suggests a more long-standing process. Multiple layers of fibrous tissue and fibrous cap with hemosiderin-laden macrophages suggest recurrent rupture.

Medial attenuation and mild chronic inflammation may be present deep to intimal lesions. It is important to evaluate regions away from atherosclerotic plaques when considering the possibility of a concurrent arteritis.

PROGNOSIS

Atherosclerosis is classically considered a largely irreversible lesion, although medical management of underlying disease such as hypertension,

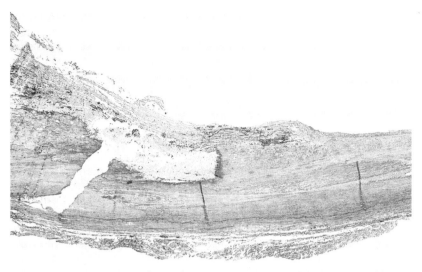

Fig. 12. Atherosclerosis. Accumulation of lipid with associated chronic inflammation and calcification can be identified in the intima of vessels involved by atherosclerosis. The underlying media may be attenuated, and sometimes even necrotic, and the adventitia may show fibrosis. It is for these reasons that the features of healed vasculitis should be evaluated at sites distinct from the areas of atherosclerotic plaque. Decalcified section, H&E stain.

hyperlipidemia, hypercholesterolemia, chronic inflammation/metabolic syndrome, and diabetes mellitus can help slow progression. Statin therapy can also lead to plaque remodeling, with increased thickness of the fibrous cap, and even modest regression of the atherosclerotic burden.[11] Occlusion secondary to progressive insidious plaque stenosis may require surgical intervention (eg, in carotid artery stenosis). Unstable plaque disease may warrant stenting and/or anti-platelet therapies to prevent infarction (eg, in coronary artery disease).

THROMBECTOMIES, EMBOLECTOMIES, AND ENDARTERECTOMIES

Specimens removed from within a vessel lumen are often not of significant diagnostic value a priori; nevertheless, these should be evaluated to ensure that no other disease process is overlooked. Thus, emboli should be evaluated for thrombotic, mycotic, neoplastic, or other origin. Endarterectomies will often contain small amounts of vessel wall, and histopathology can therefore aid in assessing adequacy and in ruling out underlying pathologies.

GROSS ASSESSMENT

The nature of the material received should be described, noting any layering of thrombi, consistency of any tissue that may represent neoplasm

(eg, myxoma or metastatic tumor), the presence of pus or necrosis that can suggest infection, and the presence or absence of calcification. Any attached vessel wall should be identified and described. Sections should be taken so as to include a cross section of vessel wall adjacent to the primary pathology. Where possible, a complete cross section of the vessel lumen is ideal. Decalcification should be used as appropriate.

MICROSCOPIC FEATURES

Layering of fibrin (so-called lines of Zahn) suggests thrombus that formed under flow conditions (**Fig. 13**, upper panel). Peripheral granulation-like

Key Considerations
THROMBECTOMIES, EMBOLECTOMIES, AND ENDARTERECTOMIES

1. Proper identification of material removed from a vessel lumen is essential to guiding therapy.

2. Emboli can be of thrombotic, infectious, neoplastic, or other origin.

3. Thrombi can be classified as unorganized, organizing, or organized based on histologic appearance, although these do not correspond perfectly with the age of the thrombus.

Fig. 13. Thrombosis. Early thrombi will show layers of blood cells and fibrin; if these form under conditions of flow, the fibrin will layer out into so-called lines of Zahn, reflecting alternating platelet-rich and fibrin/erythrocyte-rich zones (*upper panel*). With time, the clot will begin to organize into the underlying tissue, eg, vessel wall, with chronic inflammation and microvascular proliferation similar to granulation tissue, typically with hemosiderin deposition (*middle panel*). Eventually, fibrosis and well formed microvasculature will replace the thrombus (*lower panel*), often with foci of hemosiderin-laden macrophages. H&E stains.

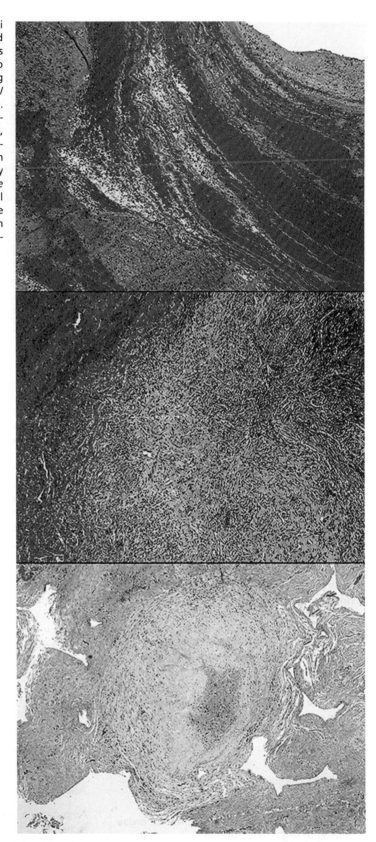

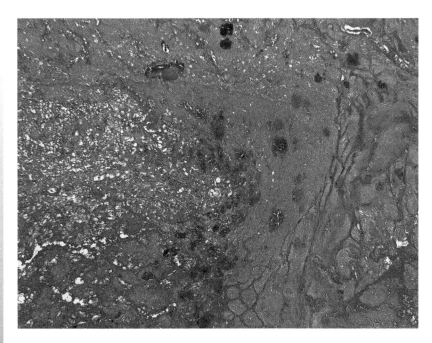

Fig. 14. Septic embolus. While appearing to be an unorganized, laminated thrombus, this embolus was found to contain plaques of bacteria, confirmed on special stains to be Gram-positive cocci. H&E stain.

changes and fibroblast proliferation suggest organization of thrombi of durations of days to over a week (see **Fig. 13**, middle panel). Fibrous replacement, often on an intimal surface and often with a myxoid quality, with multiple hemosiderin-laden macrophages suggests a fully organized remote thrombus (older than several weeks; **Fig. 14**, lower panel). Thromboemboli can retain features of the site in which they originally formed. It is also important to evaluate the endothelium and vessel wall attached to a thrombus to see if any associated pathology, eg, inflammation or infection, might be present as an explanation for the event.

Infected emboli will typically exhibit a large number of neutrophils, often with necrotic tissue debris, and even microorganisms identifiable by special stains (see **Fig. 14**).

Tumors may lack the classic features of a thrombus and instead appear very cellular. One important exception to this is that of embolized cardiac myxomas, which will have a myxoid appearance with a large number of fibroblast-like cells and small vessels, mimicking an organizing thrombus. The presence of myxoma cells, that is, angulated multinucleated cells classic to this lesion, can help in diagnosis.

Other types of emboli include fat embolism, recognizable as adipose tissue and/or bone marrow elements lodged in the vessel, and iatrogenic embolism, most commonly identified as foreign material introduced during a medical procedure.

Endarterectomies will be performed most commonly for atherosclerotic disease, and should be evaluated with that diagnosis in mind (see above). Carotid endarterectomies are most commonly performed to improve cerebral blood flow; coronary endarterectomy may be done to improve the ultimate flow downstream of a bypass graft anastomosis. Occlusive emboli, eg, in the pulmonary artery, may be removed as an endarterectomy specimen. In all such specimens, the presence or absence of attached fragments of media may aid the clinician in knowing if their procedure was adequate to remove all intimal or mural disease.

VASCULAR DISEASE IN OTHER SURGICAL SPECIMENS

A small number of additional specimen types have significant vascular pathology that merit brief comment.

AMPUTATIONS

Amputations are often performed on limbs for ischemic or microvascular disease; vessels from such specimens should be evaluated for the extent

Pitfall

THROMBECTOMIES, EMBOLECTOMIES, AND ENDARTERECTOMIES

! Embolic cardiac myxomas can mimic organizing or organized thrombi.

of vascular disease. The most commonly seen manifestations are intimal hyperplasia (usually due to hypertension or diabetic vasculopathy), medial hypertrophy (usually due to hypertension), atherosclerosis (associated with hyperlipidemia, hypercholesterolemia, hypertension, diabetes, chronic inflammation/metabolic syndrome, and genetic predisposition), and medial calcification (Mönckeberg's calcification, commonly associated with renal disease and, less commonly, diabetes). It may be appropriate in some cases to remove and decalcify large vessels before sectioning them.

SHUNT REVISIONS

Patients receiving dialysis often have surgical grafts, shunts, or fistulae that result in wall hypertrophy of the vein so that it can be used for repeated access. Revision of these may lead to removal of small segments of the involved vessels. These should be evaluated for integrity of the anastomoses, presence of any fibrinous debris suggesting possible infection, presence of aneurysmal dilation (common at the site of repeated cannulation), degree of arterialization (wall thickening/reorganization) of the venous component, and the presence of intimal hyperplasia (common at surgical anastomosis sites).

VEIN STRIPPING/THROMBOPHLEBITIS

Although much less common in modern medical management, surgical resection of veins involved by varicosities or inflammation/thrombosis (thrombophlebitis) can be received at the cutting bench. Such specimens should be evaluated primarily to rule out infection or evidence of more widespread disease. Pathologic findings in varicose veins are most commonly wall thinning; the specimen should be inspected for venous valve integrity, since valve thrombosis, degeneration, or malformation typically underlies this clinical condition. Thrombophlebitis will manifest with associated vessel wall inflammation (phlebitis). It is important to not confuse this finding with autoimmune vasculitis; distinguishing the two possibilities is done through evaluation of segments uninvolved by thrombus.

VASCULAR GRAFT/CONDUITS

Vascular reconstruction, eg, of aneurysms, dissections, or critical stenoses, typically will involve conduits of synthetic material such as polyesters (eg, Dacron) or protein matrix (such as CorMatrix). The specimen should be assessed grossly for integrity, signs of infection/fibrin accumulation, and evidence of thrombosis. Subsequent histologic evaluation will routinely demonstrate foreign body giant cell reaction to the prosthetic material, with variable degree of organizing thrombus. Intimal hyperplasia and scattered chronic inflammatory infiltrates are also common. Acute inflammation can suggest infection, but as prosthetic material may not exhibit classic responses to infection, there should be a low threshold for ordering special stains for microorganisms.

REFERENCES

1. Online Mendelian Inheritance in Man, OMIM®. MIM Number: 135580: "Fibromuscular Dysplasia of Arteries": last updated 9/08/2011. Available at: http://omim.org/. Accessed January 25, 2012.
2. Plouin PF, Perdu J, La Batide-Alanore A, et al. Fibromuscular dysplasia. Orphanet J Rare Dis 2007;2:28.
3. Rushton AR. The genetics of fibromuscular dysplasia. Arch Intern Med 1980;140:233–6.
4. Que YA, Moreillon P. Infective endocarditis. Nat Rev Cardiol 2011;8:322–36.
5. Breuer GS, Nesher R, Nesher G. Effect of biopsy length on the rate of positive temporal artery biopsies. Clin Exp Rheumatol 2009;27:S10–3.
6. Ypsilantis E, Courtney ED, Chopra N, et al. Importance of specimen length during temporal artery biopsy. Br J Surg 2011;98:1556–60.
7. Stacy RC, Rizzo JF, Cestari DM. Subtleties in the histopathology of giant cell arteritis. Semin Ophthalmol 2011;26:342–8.
8. Lee YC, Padera RF, Noss EH, et al. Clinical course and management of a consecutive series of patients with "healed temporal arteritis". J Rheumatol 2012;39:295–302.
9. Lie JT. Illustrated histopathologic classification criteria for selected vasculitis syndromes. American College of Rheumatology Subcommittee on Classification of Vasculitis. Arthritis Rheum 1990;33:1074–87.
10. Ross R. Atherosclerosis — an inflammatory disease. N Engl J Med 1999;340:115–26.
11. Zhou Q, Liao JK. Statins and cardiovascular diseases: from cholesterol lowering to pleiotropy. Curr Pharm Des 2009;15:467–78.

CARDIAC TUMORS

Dylan V. Miller, MD

KEYWORDS

• Cardiac tumor • Mass • Neoplasm • Malignancy • Myxoma • Sarcoma

ABSTRACT

Cardiac neoplasms and other mass-forming lesions are not commonly encountered in surgical pathology practice. Fortunately, for the most part, these fall into a small group of well-characterized and readily-recognized entities, although they are not without diagnostic dilemmas. A brief and practical synopsis of cardiac tumors is presented in this section with attention to more frequently encountered and clinically significant diagnostic challenges as well as pertinent clinical associations and prognostic information.

OVERVIEW OF CARDIAC TUMORS

Cardiac tumors are decidedly rare, but an understanding of their histopathologic classification, clinical associations, and biologic behavior is important in surgical pathology practice. Population-based and epidemiologic data are still lacking, but reports from autopsy series estimate their prevalence, among autopsied patients, to be 0.5% to 3.5% for all neoplasms involving the heart[1,2] and 0.001% to 0.05% for primary cardiac tumors.[3,4] Surgical series abound but few provide data on prevalence. Rates among the few that do are reported to range from 0.001% to 0.003% of patients undergoing cardiac surgery.[5,6] Similar prevalences are described in a small number of imaging series as well.[7,8] Based on the very low rates among these small and select subpopulations, the prevalence cardiac tumors in the general population may be even lower than these figures.

The great majority of all cardiac tumors are either metastatic to the heart or involve the heart secondarily by direct extension. Up to 5% of patients dying from cancer have cardiac metastases.[9] As the statistics above show, primary cardiac tumors are much less common, but are the primary focus of this article. 80 to 90% of primary cardiac tumors are benign.[10] The most common benign primary cardiac tumors in adults include (in descending order) myxoma, papillary fibroelastoma, rhabdomyoma, and fibroma (Table 1).[10–13] Malignant tumors are almost exclusively sarcomas.[14] The frequency of tumor types in children is slightly different (Table 2). In terms of biologic behavior, the prognosis of benign tumors is self evident and the "prognosis" section is omitted from the descriptions below. Where prognostic data are available, they will be provided for the malignant tumors.

The clinical significance of cardiac neoplasms depends on several factors. The tumor size is important as even benign tumors can be fatal if they grow large enough. Location is also key as even small tumors in critical sites (such as coronary ostia or within the cardiac conduction system) can cause death. Furthermore, left-sided tumors have systemic embolic potential whereas right-sided tumors embolize to the lungs (or rarely to the systemic circulation through a patent foramen ovale - a so-called "paradoxic" embolism). Location may also help narrow the differential diagnosis as some tumors have a propensity for certain sites (Box 1). Proximity to valve orifices also matters as polypoid or pedunculated tumors may exhibit a ball-valve or "tumor plop" effect with transient valvular occlusion (Fig. 1). Tumors situated within the ventricular myocardium are often implicated in arrhythmogenesis. Pericardial tumors often present with clinical features that mimic pericarditis

Intermountain Central Laboratory, Immunostains and Electron Microscopy, University of Utah, 5252 South Intermountain Drive, Salt Lake City, UT 84157, USA
E-mail address: Dylan.Miller@imail.org

Surgical Pathology 5 (2012) 453–483
doi:10.1016/j.path.2012.04.007

surgpath.theclinics.com

Table 1
Relative frequency of cardiac tumor types

	Burke, 1996 n = 386	Tazelaar, 1992 n = 110	Basso, 1997 n = 125	Odim, 2003 n = 29
Benign				
Myxoma	29%	73%	70%	69%
Papillary fibroelastoma	8%	6%	4%	3%
Rhabdomyoma	5%	—	3%	7%
Fibroma	5%	8%	3%	3%
Hemangioma	4%	1%	3%	—
Cystic tumor of AV node	3%	—	1%	—
Malignant				
Angiosarcoma	8%	2%	2%	—
Pleo. Sarcoma	4%	2%	—	—
Osteosarcoma	3%	1%	—	—
Leiomyosarcoma	3%	2%	2%	—
Fibrosarcoma	2%	—	2%	3%
Lymphoma	2%	—	—	—

Data from Refs.[10–12,14,22,35]

and pericardial constriction, though effusion, hemorrhage, and tamponade are also possible (Fig. 2). Clinical imaging by echocardiography, ECG-gated CT/MRI, and PET scan has progressed significantly in recent years. These studies are invaluable in characterizing the location, relation to vital structures, and, to some extent, the tissue characteristics of cardiac tumors, though histopathology remains the definitive means for diagnosis.[15,16]

Table 2
Frequency of primary cardiac tumors by age

Children	
Rhabdomyoma	35%
Fibroma	25%
Sarcoma	15%
Myxoma	10%
Teratoma	5%
Other	10%
Adults	
Myxoma	40%–50%
Fibroelastoma	15%
Rhabdomyoma	10%
Sarcoma	5%–10%
Fibroma	5%
Lymphoma	1%
Other	10%–15%

Box 1
Anatomic distribution of various primary cardiac tumors

Right atrium
    Angiosarcoma (80%–90% of cases)
Left atrium
    Myxoma (70%–80% of cases)
    Osteosarcoma/Pleomorphic sarcoma (>99% of cases)
Valves
    Papillary Fibroelastoma (>90% of cases; L > R)
    Myxoma (~10% of cases)
Ventricles
    Fibroma (>95% of cases)
    Rhabdomyoma (60% of cases)

Fig. 1. Echocardiographic appearance of a tumor causing "ball-valve" effect. Two-chamber view of a left atrial mass (myxoma) above the mitral annulus.

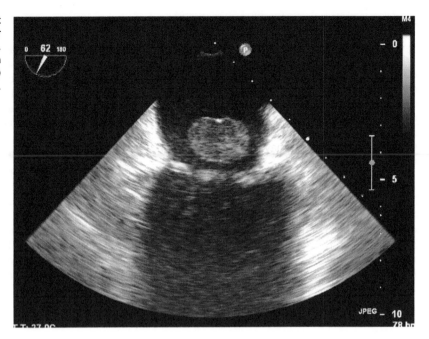

Fig. 2. Angiosarcoma with extensive pericardial involvement. Short-axis section through the ventricles at autopsy, with pericardium attached. Angiosarcoma encircling the heart and obliterating the inferior right ventricle. (*Courtesy of* William D. Edwards, MD)

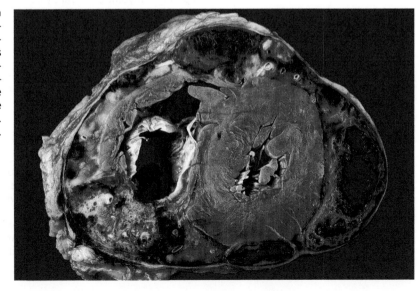

BENIGN PRIMARY CARDIAC NEOPLASMS

MYXOMA

Cardiac myxoma is the most common primary cardiac neoplasm. These tumors are thought to derive from pluripotent mesenchyme of the endocardium.[17,18] They occur at almost any age, either sporadically or as part of the Myxoma (Carney) Complex (Table 3), and may arise within any of the cardiac chambers.[3]

Gross Features of Myxoma

Deriving from the Greek for mucus (*myxa*), the gross appearance of these tumors is typically soft and gelatinous. They are often heterogenous and may contain firmer fibrous areas as well as hemorrhage (Fig. 3). An apparent stalk, typically with a patch of endocardium representing the surgical margin can usually be identified (although determining the margin status is usually unnecessary).

While any chamber can be involved, the great majority of myxomas occur in the left atrium, specifically arising from the oval fossa. Other locations as well as multifocality should raise suspicion for Myxoma (Carney) Complex.

Microscopic Features of Myxoma

The diagnostic histopathologic features of myxoma are cords and syncytia of "myxoma" cells that characteristically form rings around the small delicate vessels in the tumor (Fig. 4). The cells can be stellate or fusiform and are calretinin positive, in contrast to the vascular cells (Fig. 5). Because of their pedunculated growth, loose stroma, and continual trauma from motion of the beating heart, hemosiderin,

Table 3
Syndromes associated with cardiac tumors

	Myxoma (Carney) Complex	Tuberous Sclerosis	Basal Cell Nevus (Gorlin) Syndrome	Familial Paraganglioma (Type 4)
Clinical features	Myxomas and pigmented lesions of skin, endocrine dysfunction, benign breast and testicular tumors	Intracranial hamartomas, facial angiofibromas, subungual fibromas, renal angiomyolipomas lymphangio-myomas, and cardiac rhabdomyomas	Autosomal dominant with jaw tumors, skin cysts, basal cell carcinomas of the skin, and rarely cardiac fibromas	Multiple paragangliomas at multiple sites with variable physiologic sequelae (hypertension, other endocrine abnormalities)
Associated cardiac tumors	Myxoma	Rhabdomyoma	Fibroma	Paraganglioma
Gene defect	17q23–24 (PRKAR1A) 2p16 (Carney's locus)	9q34 (TSC1) 16p13.3 (TSC2) 12q14 (TSC3)	9q22.3 (PTCH)	1p36.13 (SDHB)
Inheritance mode	Autosomal dominant	Autosomal dominant	Autosomal dominant	Autosomal dominant
Strength of association	5% of all myxomas occur in patients with syndrome ~80% of patients with this syndrome develop cardiac myxomas	50% of all rhabdomyomas occur in patients with syndrome 25% of adults, 60% of children, and >90% of infants with syndrome have rhabdomyomas	<5% of all cardiac fibromas are associated with syndrome <10% of patients with syndrome develop cardiac fibromas	Case reports

Fig. 3. Gross appearance of cardiac myxoma. Fresh (but fragmented) and fixed cut surface of 2 different atrial myxomas. Arrows indicate the stalks and atrial attachments. Both show a soft gelatinous texture with hemorrhagic areas.

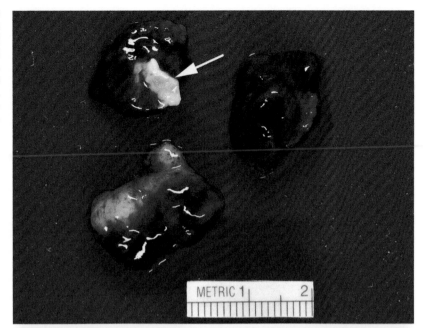

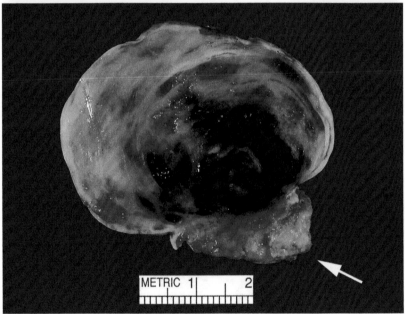

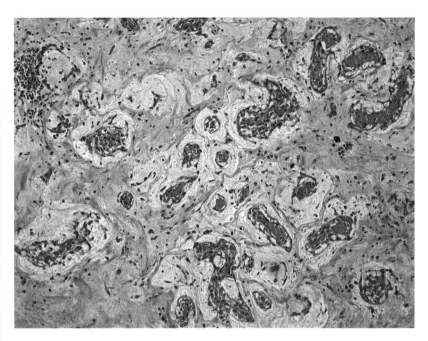

Fig. 4. Microscopic appearance of cardiac myxoma. Photomicrograph showing abundant loose myxoid matrix with rings of myxoma cells surrounding delicate vessels. There is also hemosiderin (*middle right*) and extramedullary hematopoiesis (*upper left*) (H&E ×200).

Gamna-Gandy bodies (iron encrusted elastic fibers), extravasated blood, calcification and scattered inflammatory cells are commonly seen. A diverse array of heterologous elements may be seen within myxomas, including: gland-like or squamous epithelium, cartilage, bone, thymus, and thyroid (Fig. 6).[19] Extramedullary hematopoiesis is also curiously common. Any myxoma has embolic

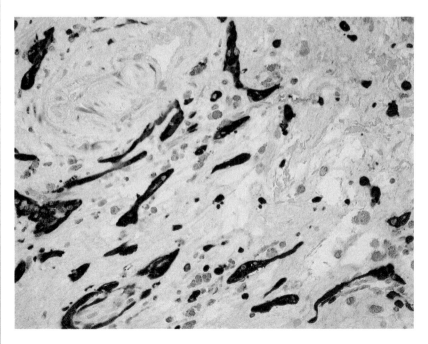

Fig. 5. Calretinin staining in cardiac myxoma. Photomicrograph showing strong cytoplasmic staining for calretinin in the myxoma cells (×400).

Fig. 6. Heterologous elements in cardiac myxoma. Photomicrographs of myxomas with osseus elements (*upper panel*, H&E, ×40) and glandular epithelium (*lower panel*, H&E, ×100).

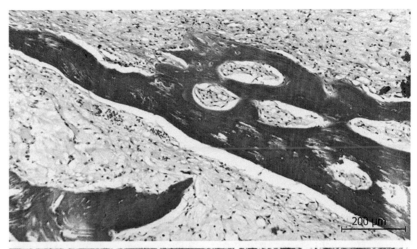

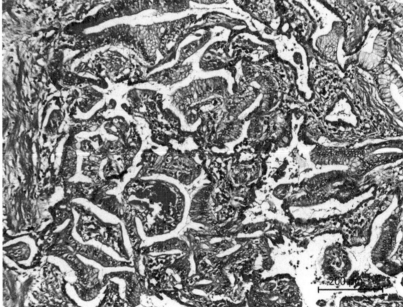

Differential Diagnosis
Myxoma

- Organizing thrombus: Myxomas were initially thought by many to be clots with exuberant organization. Myxomas with extensive (even organizing) hemorrhage can be mistaken for clots and mural thrombi with extensive granulation tissue, loose collagen, and papillary endothelial hyperplasia may mimic myxoma (Table 4).

- Papillary fibroelastoma: The globular nature and soft consistency of collapsed papillary fibroelastoma may appear grossly similar to myxoma and, without an elastic stain, the abundant loose matrix of papillary fibroelastoma microscopically resembles that seen in myxoma (see Table 4).

- Sarcomas with myxoid features: Several sarcomas may display prominent myxoid features, but typically have more cytologic atypia and mitotic activity and lack myxoma cells.

potential, but some develop frond-like projections (**Fig. 7**) and are particularly prone to embolization.[20] In such cases, myxoma emboli may be seen in vessels of the brain, kidneys, coronary arteries, and extremities[21] and may begin to grow within vessels in those distant sites. Reactive atypia may also be impressive in myxoma cells, but true malignant behavior has not been convincingly demonstrated.[22]

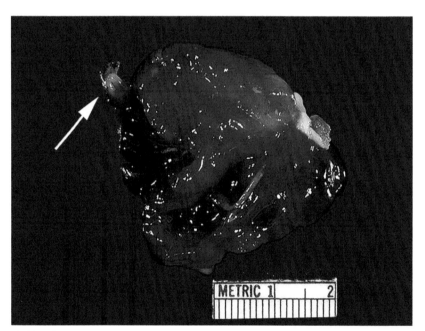

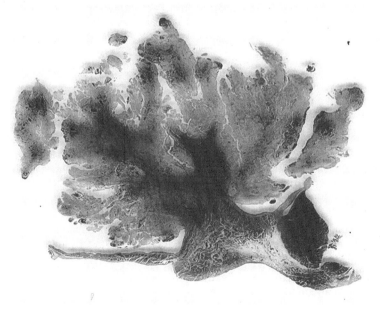

Fig. 7. Cardiac myxoma with frond-like projections. Fresh myxoma with frond-like projections (*arrow*) prone to embolization (*upper panel*) with a photograph of the corresponding H&E stained glass slide (*lower panel*).

Table 4
Features distinguishing myxoma from its main mimics

	Myxoma	Organizing Thrombus	Papillary Fibroelastoma
Gross appearance	Usually round, pedunculated	Usually sessile or more broadly tethered	Multiple fronds projecting from central core (sea anemone-like)
Histologic hallmarks	Rings of cells around vessels	Hobnail/hyperplastic endothelium without outer rings of cells	Largely devoid of vessels
Immunophenotype	Calretinin +	Calretinin −	Calretinin −
Stroma/matrix	Loose myxoid connective tissue	Variable, loose connective tissue only in organizing areas	Dense elastic tissue-rich cores
Extramedullary hematopoiesis	Yes	Rarely	No
Heterologous elements	Glandular and mesenchymal	Absent	Absent
Location	Left atrium most common (oval fossa), rarely arise from valves	Right atrium and atrial appendages, valves	Left sided valves (aortic > mitral >> tricuspid and pulmonary)

Sarcomas with myxoid features occur in the heart, but do not show other features of myxoma.

Pattern Recognition in Myxoma

- Ringing of small vessels by "myxoma cells" (calretinin positive stellate to plump spindle cells), as well as cords and syncytia of myxoma cells.
- Hematopoietic and heterologous elements.

PAPILLARY FIBROELASTOMA

Papillary fibroelastoma (PFE) is also thought to arise from pluripotent progenitor cells in the endocardium and is by most accounts the second most common primary cardiac tumor.

Gross Features of Papillary Fibroelastoma

PFEs usually arise on cardiac valves. They are composed of a thick central stalk from which emanate innumerable fine frond like projections (Fig. 8). The sea anemone-like fronds can be best appreciated when the gross specimens are suspended in clear liquid (Fig. 9). Their size ranges from a few mm to usually smaller than 5 cm. 90% occur on valves (including tendinous cords) with the left sided valves predominating (although this may represent a selection bias among surgically resected cases).[23] A form of "secondary" PFE also occurs with some frequency on diseased

(particularly rheumatic) valves (Fig. 10). Embolic complications occur, occasionally from fracturing of the fronds, but more often because of surface thrombus formation.

Differential Diagnosis and Diagnosis
PAPILLARY FIBROELASTOMA

- Lambls' excrescence: Essentially identical grossly and microscopically, but on a much smaller scale (less than 3 mm) and essentially confined to the closing edges of semilunar valve leaflets (Fig. 13) (especially at Ariantus' nodules of the aortic valve).

- Myxoma with frond-like projections: The architecture of some myxomas may loosely resemble PFE, but these myxomas will still show typical myxoma cells and lack the abundant elastic content of PFE. Myxomas rarely arise from valves.

- Thrombus: Thrombosis may occur at the surface of PFEs and then propagate to engulf the entire lesions. Valvular and other thrombi should be examined careful so as not to overlook this phenomenon. While vegetations are often in the clinical differential diagnosis, these are easily distinguished from PFE pathologically.

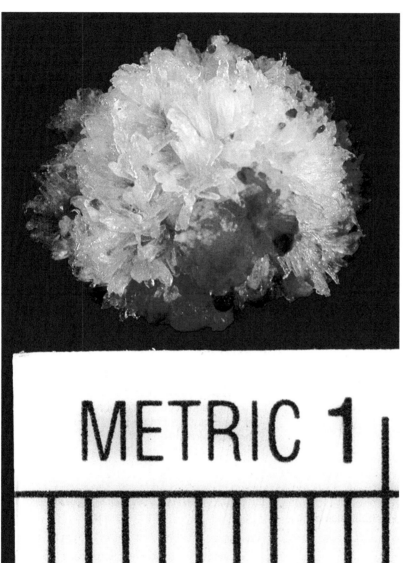

Fig. 8. Gross appearance of papillary fibroelastoma. Fixed papillary fibroelastoma showing numerous sea-anemone like fronds. The stalk is toward to the bottom of the frame.

Fig. 9. Gross appearance of papillary fibroelastoma (suspended in clear liquid). Suspending in clear liquid separates the fronds and highlights the intricate architecture of each. This can be helpful in separating myxoma from papillary fibroelastoma grossly.

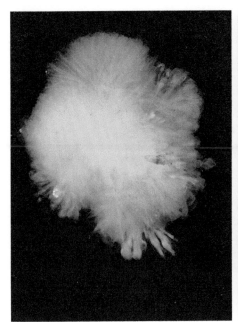
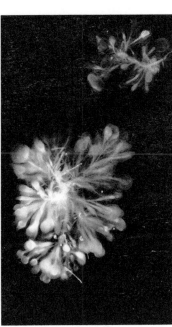

Fig. 10. Secondary papillary fibroelastoma arising on a rheumatic valve. Fixed anterior mitral leaflet with severe fusion and fibrosis of the tendinous cords and multiple "secondary" fibroelastomas. (*Courtesy of* William D. Edwards, MD)

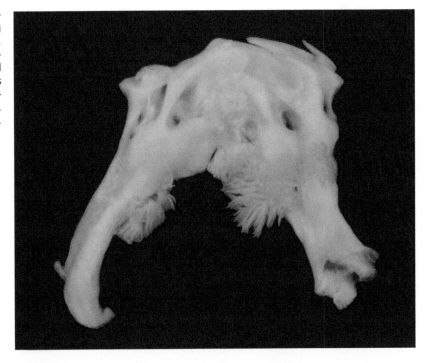

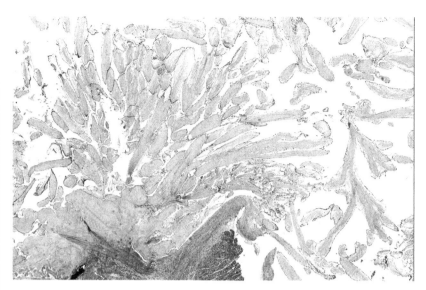

Fig. 11. Microscopic appearance of papillary fibroelastoma. Photomicrograph showing the papillary fronds radiating from a central core. The stalk and resected endomyocardium are seen in the lower middle (H&E, ×40).

Microscopic Features of Papillary Fibroelastoma

The histopathologic appearance of PFE is readily apparent, with multiple papillary fronds (Fig. 11) with predominantly avascular elastin-rich cores lined by flattened endothelium (Fig. 12). Staining for elastic tissue and endothelial antigens (CD31, CD34, FVIIIRA, etc.) can be used to highlight these components, but are rarely necessary for diagnosis.

Pattern Recognition in Papillary Fibroelastoma

- Sea anemone-like fronds composed of elastic-rich cores with endothelial lining, branching from a thick central stalk.

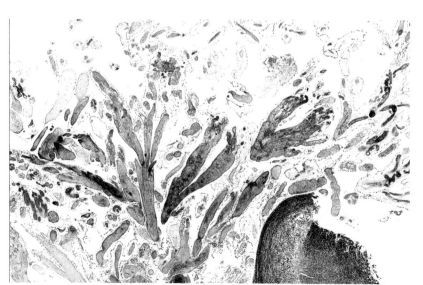

Fig. 12. Microscopic appearance of papillary fibroelastoma. Photomicrograph of the same tumor block as Fig. 11 stained for elastic tissue (*black*). The frond centers are rich in elastic tissue (Elastic Stain, ×40).

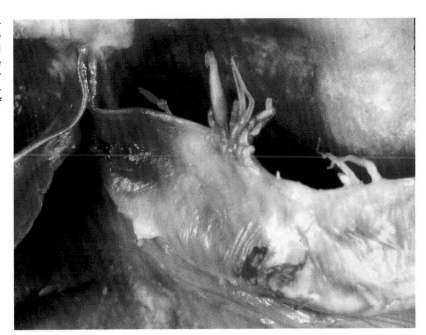

Fig. 13. Lambl excrescence. Fixed aortic valve (in situ) showing 3 small lesions with frond-like projections. The center lesion is nearest to Ariantus' nodule. (*Courtesy of William D. Edwards, MD*)

RHABDOMYOMA

Rhabdomyoma is a benign tumor of myocyte lineage that is the most common primary cardiac tumor of childhood and infancy. Most cases are associated with Tuberous Sclerosis Complex (TSC). Conversely, at least of third of patients with TSC have cardiac rhabdomyoma and 90% of those that do have multiple tumors.[24] Their clinical significance depends, as mentioned above, on the size and location of the tumor(s). Rhabdomyomas are unique among cardiac tumors in that they frequently show spontaneous regression and often do not require resection.[25]

Gross Features of Rhabdomyoma

Rhabdomyomas are fleshy lesions that are white-grey to yellow in color (**Fig. 14**). They are well-circumscribed, non-infiltrative, and often appear to "shell out" or separate easily from the tumor cavities they create. They vary in size from a few millimeters to over 9 cm. Rhabdomyomas most often occur in the ventricles, though they can arise from myocardium virtually anywhere in the heart.

Microscopic Features of Rhabdomyoma

Congruent with the gross appearance, rhabdomyomas are microscopically well-demarcated from the surrounding myocardium. They are comprised of enlarged vacuolated cells, typically much larger than surrounding normal myocytes. The sarcoplasm is replete with glycogen, often to the point that only wisps of remnant myofilaments radiate out from the nucleus in a pattern aptly referred to as a "spider cell" (**Fig. 15**). If necessary, stains for glycogen (such as PAS) and contractile elements (desmin, actin, myoglobin, etc.) may be employed to confirm the nature of these cells. The nuclei of rhabdomyoma myocytes often show marked enlargement, hyperchromasia, and irregularity. The vacuoles can resemble those seen in certain storage disease, but are limited to the tumors rather than diffusely involving the myocardium.

Pattern Recognition in Rhabdomyoma

- Well-circumscribed nodules, often multiple, based in myocardium, ventricles > atria.
- Enlarged vacuolated myocytes with spider cells

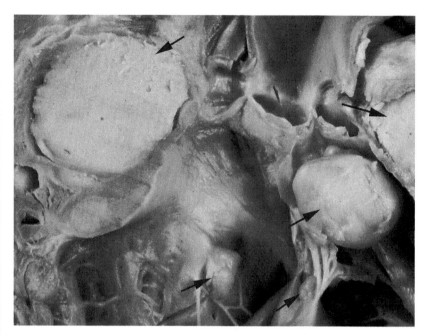

Fig. 14. Gross appearance of cardiac rhabdomyoma. Multiple rhabdomyomas (*arrows*) in a child with Tuberous Sclerosis (at autopsy). (*Courtesy of* William D. Edwards, MD)

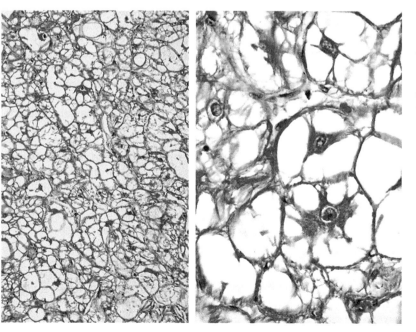

Fig. 15. Microscopic appearance of cardiac rhabdomyoma. Marked vacuolization of rhabdomyoma myocytes (*left*, H&E, ×100) with spider cells (*right*, H&E, ×400). (*Courtesy of* William D. Edwards, MD)

Fig. 16. Microscopic appearance of histiocytoid cardiomyopathy. Photomicrograph showing granular replacement of the myocyte sarcoplasm in histiocytoid cardiomyopathy. Relatively spared myocytes are seen traversing the lesion, cut in longitudinal section (H&E, ×200).

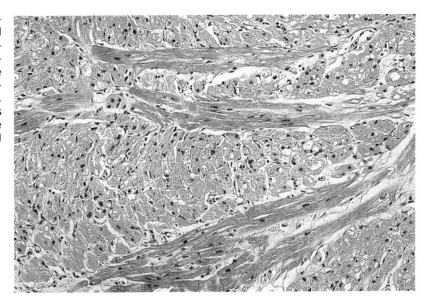

Differential Diagnosis
RHABDOMYOMA

ΔΔ

- Histiocytoid cardiomyopathy: a rare arrhythmogenic disease affecting infants, often with fatal arrhythmias. Generally small nodules resemble rhabdomyoma grossly but histologically are comprised of distended myocytes with finely granular to foamy cytoplasm without spider cells (**Fig. 16**).[26]

- Granular cell tumor: Also exceedingly rare in the heart and mostly epicardial. Typically in older patients (24 to 55 years) and identical to granular cell tumor elsewhere with uniform cells containing foamy cytoplasm, absent glycogen and expressing S-100 protein (**Fig. 17**).[27]

Fig. 17. Microscopic appearance of cardiac granular cell tumor. Photomicrograph showing rounded cells with cytoplasmic distention. The nuclei appear bland and show occasional nucleoli (H&E, ×200).

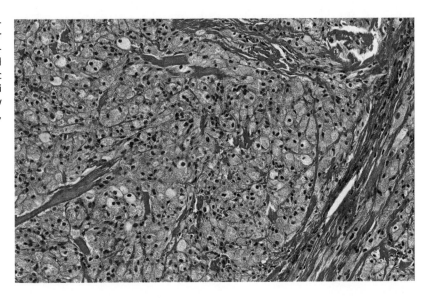

FIBROMA

Cardiac fibroma is another benign primary cardiac tumors occurring mostly in the pediatric population, though some are not detected until adulthood. Unlike rhabdomyoma, they are most often solitary and the vast majority appear to be sporadic. Only a small subset show syndromic association; namely with the Basal Cell Nevus (or Gorlin), Beckwith-Wiedeman and Sotos syndromes.[28]

Gross Features of Fibroma

Fibromas are firm, white and appear generally circumscribed, but without a capsule and are tightly adherent to the adjacent myocardium. Their cut surface is reminiscent of a uterine fibroid (Fig. 18). They occur most often in the left ventricle and ventricular septum and are usually large (around 5 cm).[28] They are almost always intramural, rather than the pedunculated forms which rhabdomyomas often assume.

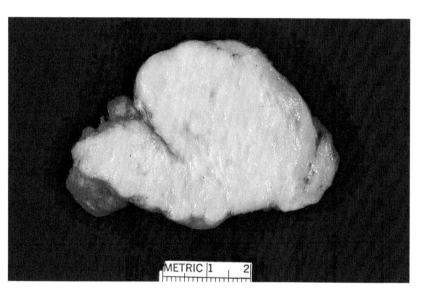

Fig. 18. Gross appearance of cardiac fibroma. Cut surface (fresh) of cardiac fibroma showing a fibrous texture and bulging surface. Wisps of enmeshed myocardium are seen at the peripheral margins.

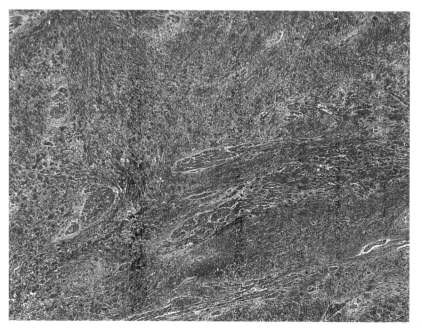

Fig. 19. Microscopic appearance of cardiac fibroma. Photomicrograph showing dense bands of collagen with fibroblasts/myofibroblasts and entrapped myocardium (taken from the edge of the lesion) (H&E, ×40).

Fig. 20. Calcifications within cardiac fibroma. Photomicrograph showing calcifications within this cardiac fibroma (H&E, ×100).

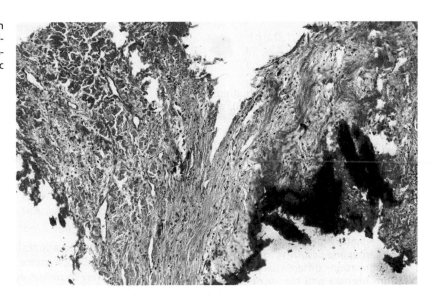

Microscopic Features of Fibroma

While grossly circumscribed, tongues of normal myocardium can be seen interdigitating with fibroma cells at the periphery of these tumors histologically (**Fig. 19**). The tumors are composed of bland myofibroblasts with varying collagen deposition surrounding them. They are devoid of myocytes, except for those entrapped at the periphery. The ratio of hyalinized collagen to fibroma cells has been reported to increase with increasing patient age.[29] Some cases show dystrophic type calcification within the tumor (**Fig. 20**). Chronic inflammation and myxoid degeneration can also be seen. The myofibroblasts stain for vimentin and SMA, but not with CD34, S100, or beta catenin.

Pattern Recognition in Fibroma

- Firm, grisly, intramural ventricular masses.
- Gross circumscription but infiltrative borders microscopically.

Fig. 21. Inflammatory myofibroblastic tumor. Photomicrograph showing a collagen-rich lesion and plump spindle cells with moderate nuclear atypia. Mixed inflammatory cells are prominent in the background (H&E, ×200).

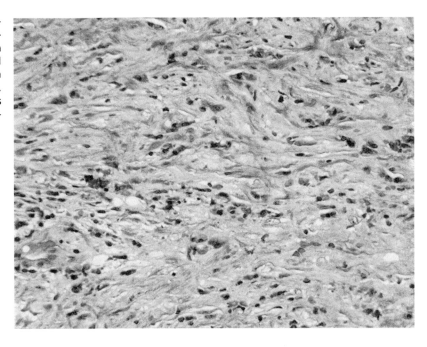

- Bland fibroblastic proliferation with hyalinized collagen (increasing with age).

HAMARTOMA OF MATURE CARDIAC MYOCYTES

Hamartoma of mature cardiac myocytes (HMCM) is a more recently described tumor, first recognized 24 years ago.[30,31] HMCM can present at any age, but the majority come to attention before age 20. There is a 4:1 male predominance.

Gross Features of Hamartoma of Mature Cardiac Myocytes

HMCM classically forms bulky intramural ventricular masses that are pale in comparison to surrounding normal myocardium and with a fibrous texture and sheen, though not as white and bulging as cardiac fibromas (Fig. 22).

Microscopic Features of Hamartoma of Mature Cardiac Myocytes

HMCM is a paradoxic lesion; despite the obvious neoplastic appearance grossly, under the microscope they show features almost identical to those of hypertrophic cardiomyopathy (Fig. 23). An important distinction, aside from the localized extent of these changes, is the presence of abnormal vessels (thick-walled arteries, and dilated venules).[32]

Pattern Recognition in Hamartoma of Mature Cardiac Myocytes

- Infiltrative mass-forming lesion of the ventricles (left > right).
- Histologically composed of benign hypertrophied myocytes with interstitial fibrosis and thick-walled arteries.

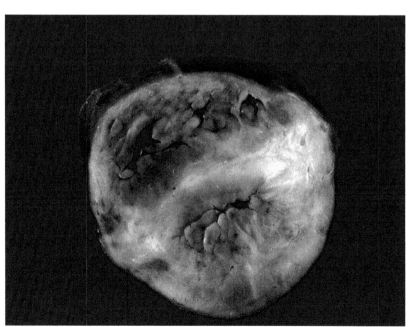

Fig. 22. Gross appearance of hamartoma or mature cardiac myocytes. Short axis section through the ventricles (fixed) showing ill-defined "grisly" masses at the anterior and inferior septum, bulging beyond the normal cardiac contours. The freewall of the left ventricle is relatively spared.

- Rhabdomyoma: While the gross appearance of rhabdomyoma is quite disparate due to its degree of circumscription, there are close histologic similarities to HMCM. True spider cells are not seen in HMCM. Additionally, rhabdomyomas are often multiple (especially in tuberous sclerosis).

- Fibroma: Fibroma may grossly resemble HMCM, but fibromas are largely devoid of myocytes whereas HMCM is comprised almost entirely of them.

- Hypertrophic cardiomyopathy: Hypertrophic cardiomyopathy often shows asymmetric involvement of the ventricles, but does not form a discrete mass. Unlike HMCM, myocardium involved by hypertrophic cardiomyopathy is identical in color and texture to the rest of the myocardium.

- Sarcoma: The grossly infiltrative appearance and bizarre hypertrophied myocyte nuclei may raise the question of sarcoma, but HMCM lacks mitotic activity, necrosis, and other features of high grade malignancy.

HEMANGIOMA AND LYMPHANGIOMA

Cardiac hemangiomas and lymphangiomas are benign vascular neoplasms similar to those occurring elsewhere in the body. Hemangiomas are much more common, accounting for roughly 5% of all benign primary tumors in the heart.[33] Lymphangiomas are exceedingly rare and often arise in the pericardium.[34,35] Both are typically asymptomatic; discovered incidentally on imaging studies performed for other indications or at autopsy.

Gross Features of Hemangiomas and Lymphangiomas

These lesions can occur anywhere in the heart. Hemangiomas are rare in the pericardium, but lymphangiomas are common there. They are generally well circumscribed and have a spongy texture (**Fig. 24**). Angiomas may be filled with blood and lymphangiomas with lymph or chylous fluid.

Microscopic Features of Hemangiomas and Lymphangiomas

Hemangiomas are classified histologically into three types: cavernous (dilated, thin-walled

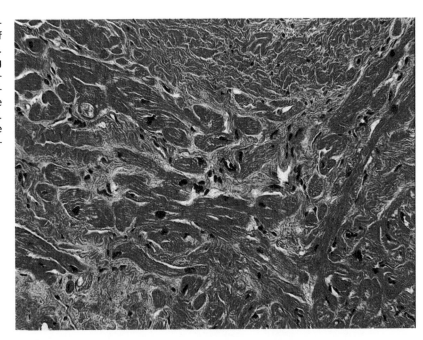

Fig. 23. Microscopic appearance of hamartoma of mature cardiac myocytes. Photomicrograph showing marked myocyte hypertrophy and interstitial fibrosis, with an appearance of "disarray" (H&E, ×400). No such changes were seen elsewhere in the uninvolved myocardium.

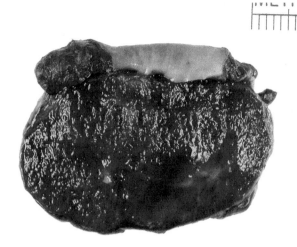

Fig. 24. Gross appearance of cardiac hemangioma. Fresh hemangioma from the right atrium (atrial septum attachment toward the top) showing a soft spongy texture and bloody appearance.

vessels), capillary, (capillary-size proliferation of vessels) and arteriovenous (malformed arteries and veins). They often have combined features though the cavernous and capillary types predominate (Fig. 25). Lymphangiomas are more cystic and may contain lymphoid aggregates and primary lymphoid follicles. The lining cells of lymphangiomas may be distinguished from hemangioma by expression of podoplanin and from mesothelial cells by absent keratin staining.

Pattern Recognition in Hemangiomas and Lymphangiomas

- Well-circumscribed lesions comprise of bland vascular spaces of varying size.

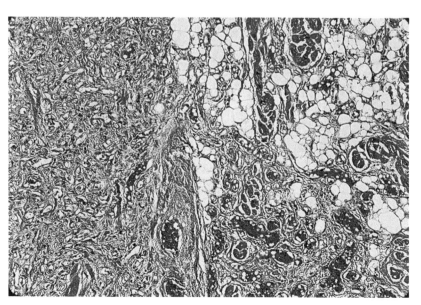

Fig. 25. Microscopic appearance of cardiac hemangioma. Photomicrograph showing capillary hemangioma pattern with proliferating capillary sized vessels (*left*) merging into the myocardium and fat (*right*) (H&E, ×100).

- Angiosarcoma: As a rule, this lesion is infiltrative at the periphery and demonstrates inter-anastomosing vascular channels and prominent cytologic atypia.

- Blood cyst: As the name implies these uniloc-ular lesions simply contain blood and do not show proliferative vascular spaces. They almost exclusively involve the atrioventricular valves (Fig. 26).

- Cystic tumor of the atrioventricular node: This lesion may superficially resemble lymphangioma. The conduction pathways in the heart are rich in lymphatics. However, cystic tumor of the atrioventricular node is not of vascular origin.

Fig. 26. Valvular blood cyst. Fixed tricuspid valve specimen showing a collapsed blood cyst after surgical excision.

LIPOMATOUS HYPERTROPHY OF THE INTERATRIAL SEPTUM

Lipomatous hypertrophy of the interatrial septum of is not a neoplasm, but unfortunately can be mistaken for one clinically. This mass-forming process in the atrial septum results from a developmental aberrancy with entrapment of fat in the septum during embryologic infolding. It is typically detected in patients over age 50 and is more common in women. It is most often asymptomatic, but may cause atrial arrhythmias and in extreme cases superior vena cava obstruction. Resection is usually not necessary, but lipomatous hypertrophy of the interatrial septum can be mistaken clinically for cardiac tumors and received as surgical specimens in pathology.

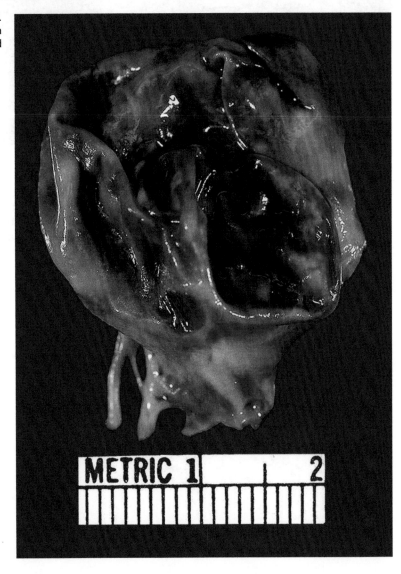

METRIC 1   2

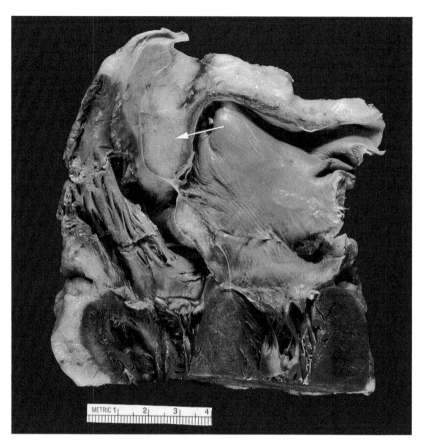

Fig. 27. Gross appearance of lipomatous hypertrophy of the interatrial septum. Hypertrophy of entrapped atrial septal fat (*arrow*), protruding into the right atrium and mimicking an atrial mass. Confinement within the septum gives the illusion of encapsulation, but there is no capsule microscopically

Gross Features of Lipomatous Hypertrophy

The "mass" formed by lipomatous hypertrophy is usually more prominent in the right atrium. The limbus portion of the fossa ovalis is typically most affected (**Fig. 27**). The gross appearance is the same as fatty tissue anywhere, though there may be fibrous trabeculae and red-brown flecks of entrapped myocardium as well.

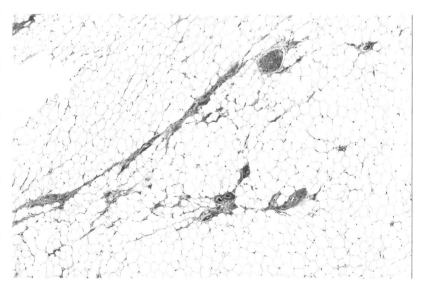

Fig. 28. Microscopic appearance of lipomatous hypertrophy of the interatrial septum. Mature adipose tissue with entrapped vessels and hypertrophied cardiomyocytes. The myocyte nuclear atypia may be dramatic, mimicking sarcoma cells, but entirely lack malignant potential (H&E, ×200).

Microscopic Features of Lipomatous Hypertrophy

Microscopically, there is no capsule and both mature and brown fat can be seen. Isolated and grouped atrial myocytes may be present and show marked hypertrophic changes (**Fig. 28**). These should not be mistaken for malignant sarcoma cells.

Pattern Recognition in Lipomatous Hypertrophy

- Mass-forming hypertrophic fat within the atrial septum, usually protruding into the right atrium.
- Benign mature fat (and/or brown fat), with entrapped myocytes, thick-walled vessels, and nerve twigs.

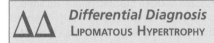

Differential Diagnosis
LIPOMATOUS HYPERTROPHY

- Cardiac Lipoma: Also composed of benign mature fat, and also may contain entrapped myocytes, but location (lipomas are usually epicardial or associated with valves) and encapsulation differentiate true lipomas from lipomatous hypertrophy of the interatrial septum.

CYSTIC TUMOR OF THE ATRIOVENTRICULAR NODE

This rare lesion demonstrates benign behavior, but its proximity to critical conduction pathways is such

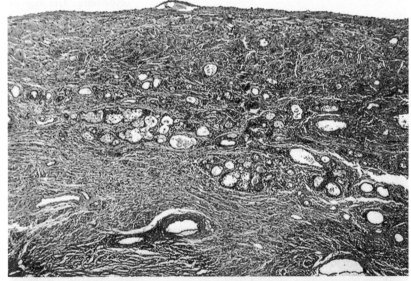
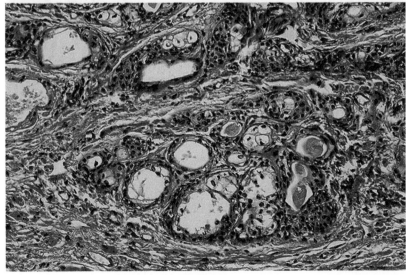

Fig. 29. Cystic tumor of the atrioventricular node. Photomicrographs showing multiple nests of cystic proliferations beneath the endocardium of the tricuspid annulus (*upper*, H&E, ×40). The cysts are lined by squamoid cells with varied but cytologically benign features (*lower*, H&E, ×200).

that it may cause sudden cardiac death. Its lineage remains somewhat cryptic and early reports describe this lesion as mesothelioma, lymphangioendothelioma, endodermal inclusion, or hamartoma. Recent work demonstrates recapitulation of a pattern seen in solid cell nests of the thyroid, suggesting they may represent ultimobranchial heterotopia.[36] Because of their ominous prognosis, surgical excision (requiring lifelong pacemaker placement) is recommended if these are detected on clinical imaging.

Gross Features of Cystic Tumor

This lesion typically shows small multilocular cysts in the vicinity of the atrioventricular node, His bundle and bundle branches. It may not be visible from the endocardial surface of the heart and requires sectioning through the infero-medial tricuspid annulus.

Microscopic Features of Cystic Tumor

Histologically, cystic tumor at the atrioventricular node shows solid nests and cystic structures lined by squamous-like cells and rare intermixed neuroendocrine cells. The cysts contain a clear to mucoid material and mucinous, ciliated, goblet and transitional type cells may also be present in the lining (Fig. 29). The cells express CK7, but not CK20, and also stain positive for EMA and CEA.

Differential Diagnosis and Diagnosis
CYSTIC TUMOR

- There are very few if any lesions that mimic this in terms of location and histopathology.

Pattern Recognition in Cystic Tumor

- Cystic and solid cell nests with mixed, but predominantly squamous-like cells.

PARAGANGLIOMA

Another exceeding rare primary cardiac neoplasm, similar in most respects to paragangliomas elsewhere. The age of reported patients ranges from 15 to 60 years with equal sex distribution and there is frequent association with the familial paraganglioma syndrome. Approximately half of the tumors are "functional", causing hypertension and other symptoms similar to pheochromocytoma (adrenal paraganglioma). The cells of origin are thought to be the cardiac ganglia, residing near conduction system structures in the atria (sinoatrial node) and near the atrioventricular septum. The innervation of these structures is

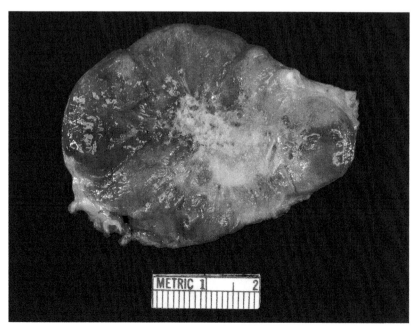

Fig. 30. Gross appearance of cardiac paraganglioma. Fresh cardiac paraganglioma showing gross lobulation, circumscribed contours, and soft texture.

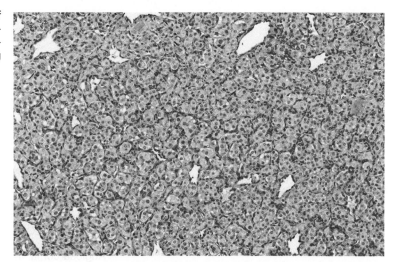

Fig. 31. Microscopic appearance of cardiac paraganglioma. Photomicrograph showing classic "Zellballen" cell nests with wrapping by sustentacular cells (H&E, ×200).

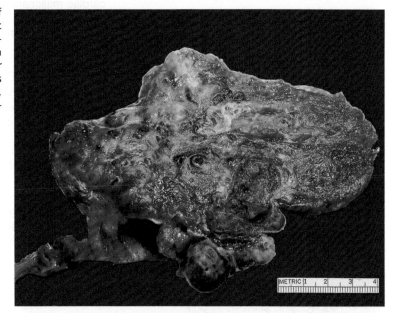

Fig. 32. Gross appearance of cardiac angiosarcoma. Right atrial angiosarcoma (fresh), resected from the right atrium (pectinate muscles at the *lower left*). The cut surface shows a highly heterogenous, soft, hemorrhagic lesion with probable areas of infarction.

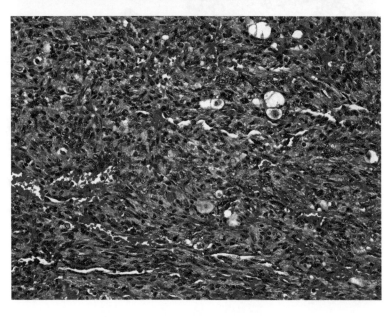

Fig. 33. Microscopic appearance of cardiac angiosarcoma. Photomicrograph showing fine interanastomosing vascular spaces with malignant-appearing spindle to epithelioid cells (H&E, ×400).

⚠️⚠️ **Differential Diagnosis and Diagnosis**
PARAGANGLIOMA

- Granular cell tumor: Grossly similar in appearance and usually situated toward the base of the heart. The tumor cells may bear some resemblance to paraganglioma, but the Zellballen architecture is lacking. Granular cell tumor cells are S100 positive, while only the sustentacular cells stain for S100 in paraganglioma.

vagal, as opposed to the sympathetic ganglion thought to give rise to aorticopulmonary paragangliomas.[37,38]

Gross Features of Paraganglioma

Typically larger (5 to 15 cm) and less well circumscribed than other sites (**Fig. 30**). Paragangliomas are almost always epicardial-based and localized to the right atrium.

Microscopic Features of Paraganglioma

The histopathology of cardiac paraganglioma is identical to what is seen at other sites as well. "Zellballen" type nests (**Fig. 31**) of neuroendocrine cells encircled by S100 positive sustentacular cells.

Pattern Recognition in Paraganglioma

- Right-sided atrial epicardial tumors.
- Typical Zellballen architecture with sustentacular cells.

MALIGNANT PRIMARY CARDIAC NEOPLASMS

These tumors will be described according to the WHO classification scheme,[39] recognizing that other nosologic systems are also in use.

ANGIOSARCOMA

Angiosarcoma is the most common primary cardiac malignancy with a peak incidence during the fourth decade. Clinical symptoms are insidious and usually absent until the tumor has reached advanced stage.

Gross Features of Angiosarcoma

Most tumors seem to arise along the right atrioventricular groove, but they can occur in any chamber as well as the pericardium. Curiously, the left atrium is the least common site (<1%). They are infiltrative into adjacent tissues and appear grossly soft and hemorrhagic (**Fig. 32**).

Microscopic Features of Angiosarcoma

The histopathology of cardiac angiosarcoma is diverse, but the majority of tumors are on the well to moderately-differentiated end of the spectrum

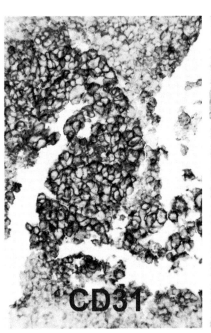
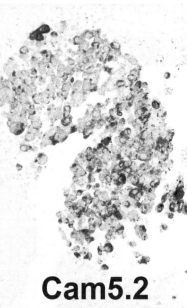

Fig. 34. Angiosarcoma immunophenotype. Photomicrographs of an angiosarcoma with epithelioid features showing strong membranous expression of CD31 (*left*) and co-expression of cytokeratin (*right*) (×400).

and commonly show epithelioid morphology (Fig. 33). The cytologically malignant cells express CD31, CD34, and FVIIIRA. Coexpression of cytokeratins and EMA is frequently seen, especially when there is epithelioid morphology (Fig. 34).

Pattern Recognition in Angiosarcoma

- Irregular inter-anastomosing vascular channels lined by cytologically malignant cells.
- High mitotic activity, hemorrhage, and necrosis.
- Expression of endothelial antigens and frequent co-expression of cytokeratins and EMA.

Prognosis in Angiosarcoma

Mortality is high with a mean survival less than 10 months. More than 80% of patients have metastases at the time of primary diagnosis.[39]

UNDIFFERENTIATED PLEOMORPHIC SARCOMA

In the WHO classification, this entity encompassed the former "malignant fibrous histiocytoma", chondrosarcoma, and osteosarcoma when they arise in the heart. Like angiosarcoma, these are aggressive lesions with frequent metastasis and dismal survival.

Gross Features of Pleomorphic Sarcoma

In contrast to angiosarcoma, most pleomorphic sarcomas arise in the left ventricle with a distribution similar to cardiac myxoma.[39] They are grossly soft, for the most part, and polypoid with a bosselated surface. Areas of necrosis and hemorrhage may be seen, but gross calcification is rare.

> ### △△ Differential Diagnosis and Diagnosis
> #### ANGIOSARCOMA
>
> - Kaposi sarcoma: There is overlap with angiosarcoma grossly and microscopically, but Kaposi sarcoma shows more spindle cell differentiation than epithelioid morphology and is HHV-8 positive.[40]
>
> - Epithelioid hemangioendothelioma: Cytologically malignant-appearing endothelial cells are focally present, though the degree of cytologic atypia is comparatively minor. Hyalinized fibrotic stroma, rather than complex vascular channels predominate in the lesion (Fig. 35). This is more often mistaken for carcinoma than angiosarcoma.
>
> - Mesothelioma: Pericardial angiosarcomas with prominent epithelioid differentiation may be mistaken for pericardial mesothelioma. Staining for calretinin and CK5 (in addition to vascular antigens) can distinguish malignant mesothelial cells from endothelial cells.

Microscopic Features of Pleomorphic Sarcoma

The histopathology is typically heterogeneous with pleomorphic cells showing spindled to epithelioid features as well as interspersed giant cells (Fig. 36). The architecture is most often storiform and areas of chondroid and/or osseous differentiation are seen in up to 15% of cases (Fig. 37).[39]

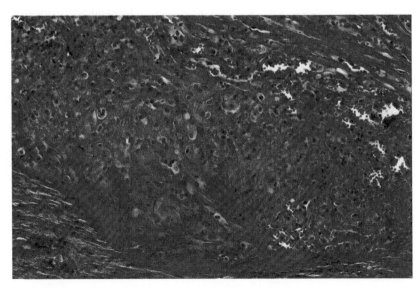

Fig. 35. Cardiac epithelioid hemangioendothelioma. Photomicrographs showing features of this low-grade malignant vascular tumor, composed of relatively more stroma and less atypical endothelial cells having more abundant cytoplasm (as compared to angiosarcoma) (×200).

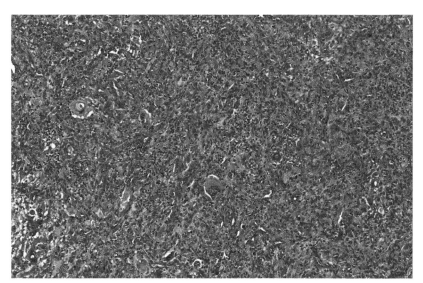

Fig. 36. Microscopic appearance of cardiac undifferentiated pleomorphic sarcoma. Photomicrographs showing highly pleomorphic cells with a vaguely storiform architecture (H&E, ×200).

This is a diagnosis of exclusion and requires absent staining for the antigens expected in leiomyosarcoma, rhabdomyosarcoma, melanoma, and neural malignancies.

Pattern Recognition in Pleomorphic Sarcoma

* Heterogeneous with markedly atypical spindled to epithelioid cells (+/- giant cells).
* Chondroid and/or osseous differentiation in up to 15% of cases.

Prognosis in Pleomorphic Sarcoma

Mortality data are sparse, but available reports from surgical series indicate median post-operative survivals between 5 and 18 months.[39]

 Differential Diagnosis and Diagnosis
PLEOMORPHIC SARCOMA

* The main entities in the differential diagnosis are other specific tissue line-of-origin sarcomas, including leiomyosarcoma, rhabdomyosarcoma, synovial sarcoma, melanoma, and malignant peripheral nerve sheath tumor. These are distinguished on the basis of their specific immunophenotypes and (increasingly) molecular diagnostics.

* Fibrosarcoma/myxosarcoma: Comparatively much more cellular, but with much less pleomorphism and prominent fascicular (even "herringbone") architecture. Tumors with abundant myxoid matrix superimposed on these changes have been called myxosarcoma (not related to myxoma) (**Fig. 38**).

LYMPHOMA

Primary cardiac lymphomas are rare, both among primary cardiac tumors and among extranodal lymphomas. The majority are high grade and form destructive lesions in the myocardium. Pericardial effusion is common, and may be the only manifestation (as in primary effusion lymphoma).

Gross Features of Lymphoma

Lymphomas may arise anywhere in the heart, forming infiltrative myocardial lesions or with polypoid projections into the chambers. They display the typical "fish-flesh" cut surface appearance (**Fig. 39**).

Microscopic Features of Lymphoma

Most primary cardiac lymphomas are of the diffuse large B-cell type (**Fig. 40**), though a variety of other types are also described. Viral mechanisms,

Differential Diagnosis and Diagnosis
LYMPHOMA

* Small round blue cell tumors: Immunohistochemical staining and/or molecular diagnostics may be required to distinguish primary cardiac lymphoma from small cell carcinoma, rhabdomyosarcoma, and other "small round blue cell" malignancies.

* Extramedullary myeloid tumor: Immunophenotyping may also be needed to separate lymphoid malignancies from myeloid lineage tumors.

Fig. 37. Pleomorphic sarcoma with osseous differentiation (formerly cardiac osteosarcoma). Photomicrographs showing a sarcoma with comparatively less cytologic atypia but formation of osteoid matrix (H&E, ×200).

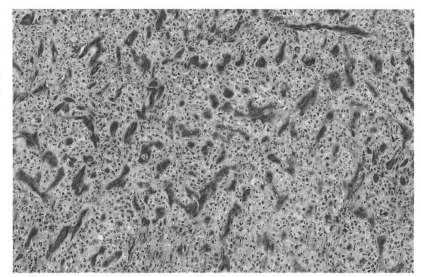

Fig. 38. Cardiac myxosarcoma. Photomicrographs showing malignant pleomorphic sarcoma with prominent myxoid extracellular matrix (H&E, ×200).

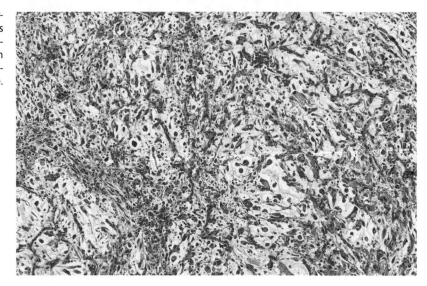

Fig. 39. Gross appearance of primary cardiac lymphoma. Primary cardiac lymphoma (fixed) with white and "fish-fleshed" appearance, destructively involving the left ventricular free wall and pericardium.

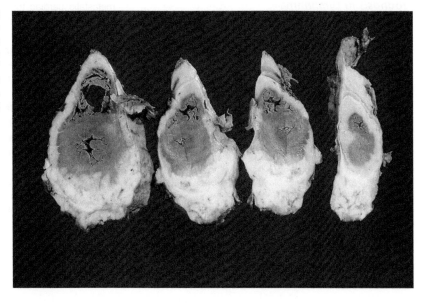

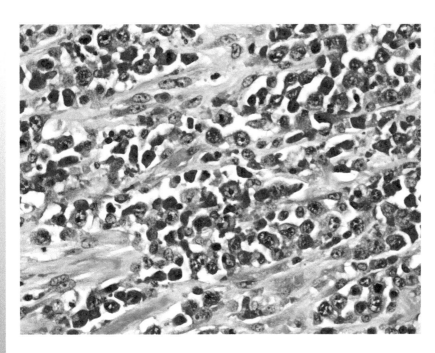

Fig. 40. Microscopic appearance of primary cardiac lymphoma. Photomicrograph showing malignant lymphocytes with "blastic" features (H&E, ×600).

particularly Epstein-Barr virus related, are increasingly recognized in these lymphoma, particularly in the immunocompromised, elderly, and when foreign material is present.[41]

Pattern Recognition in Lymphoma

- Highly cellular with monomorphic, dyscohesive cells and frequent mitoses/karyorrhectic bodies.
- Most cases are diffuse large B-cell lymphoma.

Prognosis in Lymphoma

Like the sarcomas previously discussed, primary cardiac lymphomas are often clinically silent until the late stages. Survival after diagnosis is poor with 60% mortality at less than 2 months in one study.[42]

REFERENCES

1. Reynen K. Frequency of primary tumors of the heart. Am J Cardiol 1996;77(1):107.
2. Butany J, Leong SW, Carmichael K, et al. A 30-year analysis of cardiac neoplasms at autopsy. Can J Cardiol 2005;21(8):675–80.
3. Wold LE, Lie JT. Cardiac myxomas: a clinicopathologic profile. Am J Pathol 1980;101(1):219–40.
4. Lam KY, Dickens P, Chan AC. Tumors of the heart. A 20-year experience with a review of 12,485 consecutive autopsies. Arch Pathol Lab Med 1993;117(10): 1027–31.
5. Dein JR, Frist WH, Stinson EB, et al. Primary cardiac neoplasms. Early and late results of surgical treatment in 42 patients. Thorac Cardiovasc Surg 1987; 93(4):502–11.
6. Murphy MC, Sweeney MS, Putnam JB Jr, et al. Surgical treatment of cardiac tumors: a 25-year experience. Ann Thorac Surg 1990;49(4):612–7.
7. Sutsch G, Jenni R, von Segesser L, et al. Heart tumors: incidence, distribution, diagnosis. Exemplified by 20,305 echocardiographies. Schweiz Med Wochenschr 1991;121(17):621–9 [in German].
8. Strecker T, Rösch J, Weyand M, et al. Primary and metastatic cardiac tumors: imaging characteristics, surgical treatment and histopathological spectrum: a 10-year-experience at a german heart center. Cardiovasc Pathol 2012. [Epub ahead of print].
9. Prichard RW. Tumors of the heart; review of the subject and report of 150 cases. AMA Arch Pathol 1951;51(1):98–128.
10. Burke A, Virmani R. Classification and incidence of cardiac tumors. In: Burke A, Virmani R, editors. Tumors of the heart and great vessels. Washington, DC: Armed Forces Institute of Pathology; 1996. p. 1–12.
11. Odim J, Reehal V, Laks H, et al. Surgical pathology of cardiac tumors. Two decades at an urban institution. Cardiovasc Pathol 2003;12(5):267–70.
12. Tazelaar HD, Locke TJ, McGregor CG. Pathology of surgically excised primary cardiac tumors. Mayo Clin Proc 1992;67(10):957–65.
13. Burke AP, Cowan D, Virmani R. Primary sarcomas of the heart. Cancer 1992;69(2):387–95.

14. Basso C, Valente M, Poletti A, et al. Surgical pathology of primary cardiac and pericardial tumors. Eur J Cardiothorac Surg 1997;12:730–8.

15. Buckley O, Madan R, Kwong R, et al. Cardiac masses, part 2: key imaging features for diagnosis and surgical planning. Am J Roentgenol 2011;197(5):W842–51.

16. Anavekar NS, Bonnichsen CR, Foley TA, et al. Computed tomography of cardiac pseudotumors and neoplasms. Radiol Clin North Am 2010;48(4):799–816.

17. Acebo E, Val-Bernal JF, Gómez-Román JJ. Prichard's structures of the fossa ovalis are not histogenetically related to cardiac myxoma. Histopathology 2001;39(5):529–35.

18. Kodama H, Hirotani T, Suzuki Y, et al. Cardiomyogenic differentiation in cardiac myxoma expressing lineage-specific transcription factors. Am J Pathol 2002;161(2):381–9.

19. Miller DV, Tazelaar HD, Handy JR, et al. Thymoma arising within cardiac myxoma. Am J Surg Pathol 2005;29(9):1208–13.

20. Michelena HI, Miller DV, Schaff HV. A dangerous myxoma. Cardiovasc Pathol 2010;19(6):e251–2.

21. Burke AP, Virmani R. Cardiac myxoma. A clinicopathologic study. Am J Clin Pathol 1993;100(6):671–80.

22. Burke A, Virmani R. Cardiac myxoma. In: Burke A, Virmani R, editors. Tumors of the heart and great vessels. Washington, DC: Armed Forces Institute of Pathology; 1996. p. 21–46.

23. Burke A, Tazelaar H, Gomez-Roman JJ, et al. Benign tumors of pluripotent mesenchyme. In: Travis WD, Brambilla E, Muller-Hermelink HK, et al, editors. Pathology & genetics: tumors of the lung, pleura, thymus, and heart. Lyon (France): IARC press; 2004. p. 260–5.

24. Shehata BM, Burke AP, Tazelaar H, et al. Benign tumors with myocyte differentiation. In: Travis WD, Brambilla E, Muller-Hermelink HK, et al, editors. Pathology & genetics: tumors of the lung, pleura, thymus, and heart. Lyon (France): IARC press; 2004. p. 254–9.

25. Bosi G, Lintermans JP, Pellegrino PA, et al. The natural history of cardiac rhabdomyoma with and without tuberous sclerosis. Acta Paediatr 1996;85(8):928–31.

26. Shehata BM, Patterson K, Thomas JE, et al. Histiocytoid cardiomyopathy: three new cases and a review of the literature. Pediatr Dev Pathol 1998;1(1):56–69.

27. Qi J, Yu J, Zhang M, et al. Multicentric granular cell tumors with heart involvement: a case report. J Clin Oncol 2012;30(6):e79–82.

28. Miller DV, Wang H, Wang H, et al. Beta-catenin mutations do not contribute to cardiac fibroma pathogenesis. Pediatr Dev Pathol 2008;11(4):291–4.

29. Burke AP, Rosado-de-Christenson M, Templeton PA, et al. Cardiac fibroma: clinicopathologic correlates and surgical treatment. J Thorac Cardiovasc Surg 1994;108(5):862–70.

30. Tanimura A, Kato M, Morimatsu M. Cardiac hamartoma. A case report. Acta Pathol Jpn 1988;38(11):1481–4.

31. Burke AP, Ribe JK, Bajaj AK, et al. Hamartoma of mature cardiac myocytes. Hum Pathol 1998;29(9):904–9.

32. Fealey ME, Edwards WD, Miller DV, et al. Hamartomas of mature cardiac myocytes: report of 7 new cases and review of literature. Hum Pathol 2008;39(7):1064–71.

33. Grebenc ML, Rosado de Christenson ML, Burke AP, et al. Primary cardiac and pericardial neoplasms: radiologic-pathologic correlation. Radiographics 2000;20(4):1073–103.

34. Kaji T, Takamatsu H, Noguchi H, et al. Cardiac lymphangioma: case report and review of the literature. J Pediatr Surg 2002;37(10):E32.

35. Burke A, Virmani R. Vascular tumors and tumor-like conditions. In: Burke A, Virmani R, editors. Tumors of the heart and great vessels. Washington, DC: Armed Forces Institute of Pathology; 1996. p. 79–90.

36. Cameselle-Teijeiro J, Santías RR, Nallib IA, et al. Cystic tumor of the atrioventricular node: a rare cardiac pseudoneoplastic lesion. Arch Pathol Lab Med 2010;134(11):1584–6.

37. Huo JL, Choi JC, Deluna A, et al. Cardiac paraganglioma: diagnostic and surgical challenges. J Card Surg 2012;27(2):178–82.

38. Jebara VA, Uva MS, Farge A, et al. Cardiac pheochromocytomas. Ann Thorac Surg 1992;53(2):356–61.

39. Burke AP, Veinot JP, Tazelaar H, et al. Cardiac sarcomas. In: Travis WD, Brambilla E, Muller-Hermelink HK, et al, editors. Pathology & genetics: tumors of the lung, pleura, thymus, and heart. Lyon (France): IARC press; 2004. p. 273–81.

40. Pantanowitz L, Dezube BJ. Kaposi sarcoma in unusual locations. BMC Cancer 2008;8:190.

41. Miller DV, Firchau DJ, McClure RF, et al. Epstein-Barr virus-associated diffuse large B-cell lymphoma arising on cardiac prostheses. Am J Surg Pathol 2010;34(3):377–84.

42. Chalabreysse L, Berger F, Loire R, et al. Primary cardiac lymphoma in immunocompetent patients: a report of three cases and review of the literature. Virchows Arch 2002;441(5):456–61.

EXAMINATION OF THE CARDIAC EXPLANT

Barbara A. Sampson, MD, PhD

KEYWORDS

• Cardiac • Transplant • Explant • Pathology • Dissection

ABSTRACT

Examination of cardiac explants is a challenge to the surgical pathologist. This is due to the complex anatomy of the heart, the numerous pathologies unique to the heart, and the complexities of cardiovascular interventions including the transplant procedure itself. The dissection technique described permits complete evaluation of the heart with good photographic and histologic documentation while maintaining the integrity of the specimen.

OVERVIEW OF CARDIAC EXPLANTS

Proper evaluation of cardiac explants requires a systematic approach with consideration of the possible underlying pathology before beginning the dissection. The technique to use differs between ischemic heart disease and other cardiomyopathies. Familiarity with normal cardiac anatomy, and in the case of congenital heart disease, with the anatomy of the defect(s), is of paramount importance. The technique must also allow full evaluation of surgical interventions and any related devices, full photographic and histologic documentation, retention of myocardium for any ancillary studies (such as electron microscopy or genetic testing, if applicable), and preservation of the specimen for teaching or later review.

THE TRANSPLANT PROCEDURE

During transplantation, the donor heart must be anastomosed to the recipient's native tissues. The procedure involves the following:

1. Systemic venous anastomosis to the right atrium. Originally, an atrial anastomosis was used. The procedure most commonly used today is the bi-caval anastomosis which separately anastomoses the donor and recipient superior and inferior vena cavae and preserves normal atrial anatomy.

Key Considerations
CARDIAC EXPLANT

• Explanted hearts are generally not intact.

• Prior surgical procedures must be documented.

• Coronary artery stents are common in ischemic heart disease; the stented arterial segments may require special processing (see the article by Padera elsewhere in this issue).

• Dissection of the explanted heart for ischemic heart disease should consist of transverse sections of the ventricles with the base of the heart opened along the lines of flow, similarly to the standard autopsy heart dissection.

• Histologic sections should include routine sampling and sections of all major pathology.

• Histologic aging of recent myocardial infarcts should be performed on sections of peripheral edges of infarct.

2. Transection of the recipient great arteries immediately above the valves and anastomosis to the corresponding donor vessels.
3. Transection of the recipient left atrium anterior to the pulmonary veins leaving a cusp of atrial tissue which is anastomosed to the donor atrium.

The structures absent from the explanted heart depend upon the surgical procedure used.

DISSECTION OF THE EXPLANTED HEART FOR ISCHEMIC HEART DISEASE

EVALUATION OF HEART SIZE

The first question to address is whether the heart is normal sized or enlarged. The explanted heart

Office of the Chief Medical Examiner of the City of New York, 520 First Avenue, New York, NY 10016, USA
E-mail address: BSampson@ocme.nyc.gov

Surgical Pathology 5 (2012) 485–495
doi:10.1016/j.path.2012.04.008
1875-9181/12/$ – see front matter © 2012 Elsevier Inc. All rights reserved.

weight should be recorded and approximate comparisons may be made to reference range tables previously published, keeping in mind that some heart tissue is missing from the specimen.[1] If the heart is enlarged, the external impression of which side of the heart and which chambers are involved should be noted. This will be confirmed later upon internal examination.

EXTERNAL SURFACES

Document what is received. The general shape of the heart should be noted (globular, marked hypertrophy or dilatation of the chambers), as should the relationship of the great vessels. Externally visible areas of hemorrhage or fibrosis should be noted. Adhesions and prior surgical interventions may complicate the examination.

Patients with atherosclerotic coronary disease may have had coronary artery bypass grafting before they come to transplant. Each graft must be described including type (saphenous vein vs mammary artery), origin, distal anastomosis, and patency. A comment about the integrity of the suture lines should be included. In addition, cardiac devices are commonly encountered in explanted hearts, including pacemakers, defibrillators, and ventricular assist devices (see the article by Padera elsewhere in this issue).

Finally, preliminarily examine the valves through the atria, noting any evidence of degenerative disease, thrombus, or vegetations.

CORONARY ARTERY DISSECTION

Once the external features have been documented, the dissection can continue beginning with dissection of the coronary arteries.

1. Document coronary artery dominance. Eighty percent of cases will be right dominant, defined as the right coronary artery providing the posterior descending coronary artery which supplies blood to the posterior wall of the left ventricle. Ten percent will be left dominant in which the posterior descending coronary artery arises from the left circumflex coronary artery and ten percent will be co-dominant with a posterior descending coronary artery arising from both the right coronary artery and left circumflex coronary artery.
2. The major epicardial coronary arteries should be identified (Fig. 1), removed from the heart, decalcified if necessary, and serially cross sectioned at 3 mm intervals through the entire length of the artery including all major branches (Fig. 2).
3. The degree of luminal narrowing and extent of the disease (diffuse or focal) should be noted.

4. The presence of coronary arterial thrombosis should be documented.
5. Any additional coronary artery abnormality should be documented including abnormal origin, abnormal course, aneurysms, or dissections.

Coronary artery stents are commonly encountered in ischemic heart disease (see the article by Padera elsewhere in this issue).[2]

VENTRICULAR EXAMINATION OF CARDIAC EXPLANT

Following dissection of the major coronary arteries, the myocardium must be examined. This is best accomplished by making three to four cross-sectional slices through the ventricles from the ventricular apex to the mid ventricular level, which is approximately at the level of the papillary muscles (Fig. 3A). This cross-sectional approach allows more area of the ventricular myocardium to be examined. This is especially important in cases of ischemic disease to fully evaluate the myocardium for evidence and extent of infarct. Also full thickness histologic sections of myocardium can easily be taken (see Fig. 3A, B).

The remainder of the heart should be opened along the direction of flow of blood (Fig. 4A); that is, it should be opened by cutting from the right atrium through the tricuspid valve into the right ventricle, out the pulmonary valve, then from the left atrium through the mitral valve into the left ventricle and out the aortic valve.

Detailed description of the dissection follows:

1. Using scissors, open the remaining right atrium from the area of the inferior vena cava to the tip of the right atrial appendage, looking for atrial appendage thrombi.
2. Examine the atrial septal anatomy (including the patency of the foramen ovale), coronary sinus ostium, and the connections of the inferior vena cava and superior vena cava with the right atrium (if present).
3. Open the right ventricle (see Fig. 4A1). The cut should be through the tricuspid valve annulus toward the apex through the lateral or posterior wall of the right ventricle (away from the ventricular septum).
4. Any pathology of the tricuspid valve, the right ventricular size, the thickness of the compact myocardium and any gross changes to the myocardium should be documented (see Fig. 4B).
5. Note that the wall thickness measurement should be done at the mid ventricular level in the posterior wall and should include only the compact myocardium, not the trabeculations.

Fig. 1. (*A*) Dissection of left main coronary artery and its major branches. At minimum, the left main, left anterior descending, and left circumflex arteries should be examined. (*B*) Dissection of the right coronary artery and posterior descending coronary artery. The right coronary artery gives rise to the posterior descending artery making this heart right dominant. NOTE: In this case, ventricular cross sections were made before dissection of the coronary arteries.

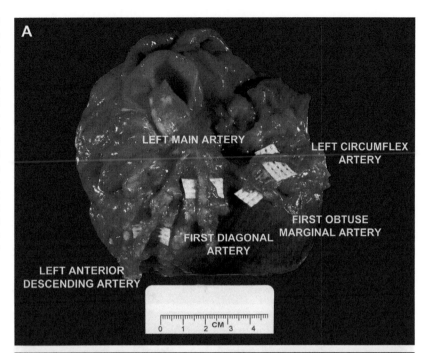

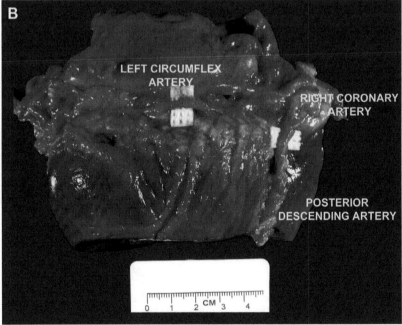

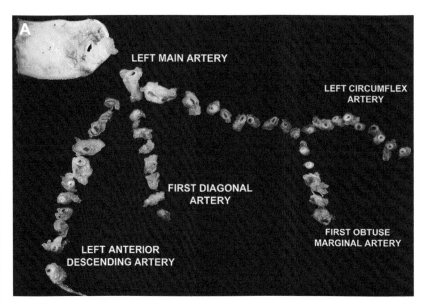

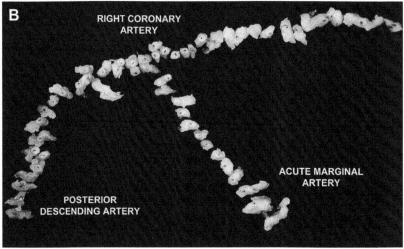

Fig. 2. (A) Sections of the left coronary artery and its branches at 3 mm intervals. This practice allows for careful examination of the degree of atherosclerosis and presence of any arterial thrombus. (B) Similar sections of the right coronary artery and its branches.

6. The right ventricular outflow tract cut should be made on the anterior aspect of the heart with the blade anterior to the anterior papillary muscle of the tricuspid valve (see Fig. 4A2). The cut goes through the pulmonary valve and into the pulmonary artery (if present), permitting complete visualization of the right ventricular outflow tract, including the perimembranous region of the ventricular septum, which is the most common site of a ventricular septal defect (see Fig. 4C).

7. Any pathology of these structures should be documented.

The dissection continues on the left side of the heart. Often in the explanted heart the left atrium is received opened. If not, it should now be opened with scissors and the atrial appendage should be examined for thrombi.

1. The left ventricle is opened along the lateral wall. The cut is made through the mitral valve between the two papillary muscles (see Fig. 4A3).

2. Annulus size, annular calcification, and pathology of the mitral valve leaflets, chordae tendineae and papillary muscles should be documented (see Fig. 4D).

Fig. 3. (*A*) Schematic depicting method for obtaining cross sections of the ventricles. LV, left ventricle; RV, right ventricle; VS, ventricular septum. (*B*) An example of a ventricular cross section showing areas of old infarct (white) in the posterior wall.

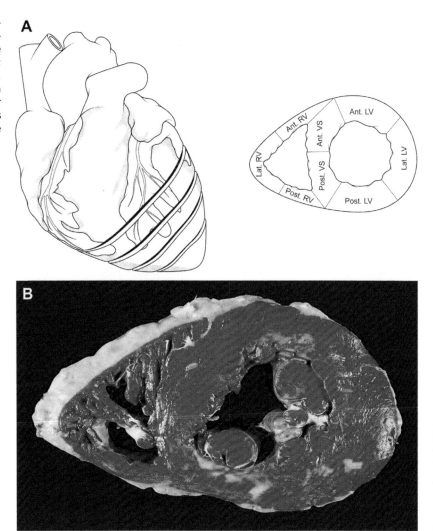

3. The appearance of the endocardium and myocardium should be documented as well as the location and extend of a recent or old myocardial infarct.

4. The thickness of compact myocardium (that is, excluding the trabeculations) of the lateral wall at the mid ventricular level should be recorded.

5. To make the left ventricular outflow incision, visualize the aortic valve, and orient the heart so that the anteroseptal wall of the left ventricle is flat on the dissecting table.

6. Place the blade immediately behind the anterolateral papillary muscle and cut through the anterior wall (see **Fig. 4**A4). This cut should only extend halfway up the left ventricular outflow tract.

7. The remainder of the incision is made by positioning the heart with the aortic aspect downward on the dissecting table.

8. Using a scalpel, extend the incision to the aortic valve (see **Fig. 4**A5).

9. When the aortic valve is visualized, reflect the pulmonary artery anteriorly and the left atrial appendage posteriorly and using a scissors, open the aortic valve through the commissure between the right and left cusps (see **Fig. 4**E).

This approach allows for examination of the aortic valve and coronary artery ostia, which should now be on either side of the incision.

Examine the shape of the ventricular septum, note whether the septum is intact, and describe

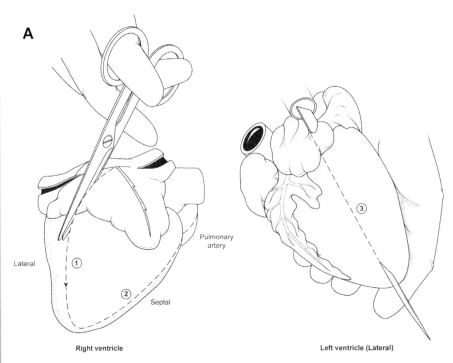

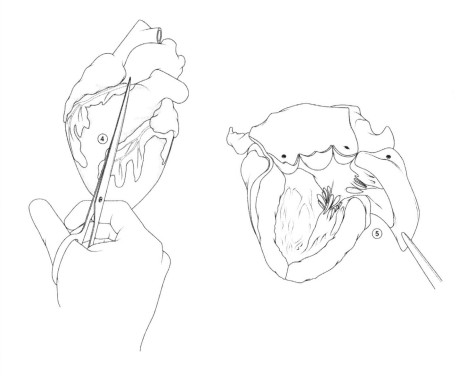

Fig. 4. (*A*) Schematic depicting opening the heart (or base of the heart) according to lines of flow.

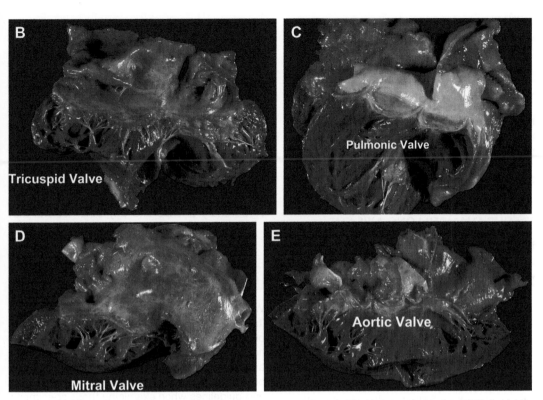

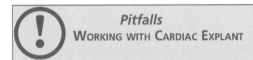

Fig. 4. (*B*) The right atrium and right ventricle have been opened to expose the tricuspid valve. (*C*) The pulmonary outflow tract has been opened to show the pulmonic valve. (*D*) The left atrium and left ventricle have been opened to show the mitral valve. (*E*) The aortic outflow tract has been opened showing the aortic valve.

the aortic valve including the number of cusps, any changes to the cusps and the presence of any lesions. The coronary artery ostia should arise centrally from their respective sinuses of Valsalva and below the sinotubular ridge.

ROUTINE HISTOLOGY OF CARDIAC EXPLANT

Examination of an explanted heart is incomplete without histology. Transmural sections of the walls of the right and left ventricle provide a good sampling of the myocardium. In addition, any lesions noted grossly should be sampled histologically. Myocardial infarcts heal from the periphery inward; therefore, when aging infarcts, sections should be taken from the peripheral edges of the infarct. Cross sections of coronary arteries demonstrating the most critical areas of narrowing should be submitted after decalcification to document the severity of the atherosclerotic disease. Eosinophilic (hypersensitivity) myocarditis is often seen in explanted hearts. It is usually considered an incidental finding related to one or more of the many drugs taken by transplant candidates.

> ## Pitfalls
> ### WORKING WITH CARDIAC EXPLANT
>
> ! Medical chart review is important in the evaluation of an explanted heart; however, the pathologist must not allow the clinical impression to constrain his objective diagnostic evaluation.
>
> ! Different cardiac pathologic conditions may have similar features, but totally different underlying etiologies and implications for family members.
>
> ! Several potentially inheritable cardiomyopathies have extensive left ventricular scarring and can be mistaken for ischemic heart disease, including but not limited to end stage hypertrophic cardiomyopathy (HCM),[3] left ventricular noncompaction and arrhythmogenic cardiomyopathy, left ventricular dominant form.[4] Each of these types of cardiomyopathies is potentially inheritable, and correct diagnosis is essential to facilitate evaluation of family members and prevent sudden death. Genetic testing may be helpful in some cases.

DISSECTION OF THE EXPLANTED HEART FOR CARDIOMYOPATHY

EXTERNAL SURFACE-GENERAL FEATURES AND HEART SIZE

The external examination is similar to that of the heart with ischemic heart disease. The major coronary arteries, if uncalcified, should then be sectioned at 3 mm intervals in situ from their origin along their entire route.

THE FOUR CHAMBER LONG AXIS CUT

After fixation, a four chamber long axis cut (apical four chamber cut) may be performed (Fig. 5A). This divides the heart longitudinally from apex to base.

1. Using a long, sharp knife, bisect the tricuspid and mitral valves, thereby bisecting the atria and ventricles. This provides an exceptional view of the myocardium and maintains the integrity of the specimen (see Fig. 5B).
2. The ventricular chambers should be assessed. Are they hypertrophied or dilated? Is there evidence of mottling, infiltrative disease, fibrosis or recent infarct? If so, document the location and extent. Photography is useful.
3. Evaluate the endocardial surface in particular. Is there evidence of an aortic outflow tract plaque, indicative of hypertrophic cardiomyopathy? Is the right ventricle replaced by fat, suggestive of arrhythmogenic cardiomyopathy?
4. The thickness of the right ventricle, septum, and left ventricle should be recorded.
5. The pulmonic and aortic valves should now be opened to fully assess these valves as well as the surgical anastomoses. This can be done from the posterior aspect of the heart so that the cut surface remains intact. Any tissue removed for ancillary studies or research should be documented.
6. Sections for histology should include at a minimum representative section of the left and right ventricles and septum.
7. Coronary arteries and any other lesions may also be submitted for histology.

EXPLANTED HEART WITH CONGENTIAL HEART DISEASE

With the success in surgical treatment of congenital heart disease, more patients are living to an older age, some eventually requiring transplantation. An exhaustive list of congenital conditions and their surgical treatment is beyond the scope of this review. Below are general considerations and guidelines when examining these specimens.

Review of the clinical history, symptoms and imaging studies may be useful before examination of the heart. If there has been previous surgical intervention, review of the operative report(s) may also be very helpful. All sutures, suture lines, and grafts should be documented before dissection.

Morphologic features and embryonic development play an important role in congenital heart disease. General knowledge and understanding of these features before dissection is essential for appropriate modification of the dissection technique. Complex congenital heart disease is often outside the realm of the surgical pathologist; consultation with a cardiac pathologist, or if not available, review with a pediatric cardiologist, may be necessary.

EXPLANTED HEART WITH VALVULAR DISEASE

Minimal modification of the usual dissection technique is required for explants with valvular heart disease. With marked aortic stenosis, one may wish to keep the left ventricular outflow tract intact. Explanted hearts may have prior valve replacement surgery or annuloplasty rings. In general, such a heart should not be opened through the prosthetic valve, but should be opened sufficiently to visualize and evaluate the valve (see the article by VanderLaan and colleagues elsewhere in this issue).

Key Considerations
DIAGNOSIS OF THE CARDIAC EXPLANT

- Accurate diagnosis of the particular cardiomyopathy is of utmost importance. Many cardiomyopathies are heritable. Communication of such a diagnosis to the physician and/or patient may have great implications for family members.

- Certain diseases may recur in the allograft (such as sarcoidosis or amyloidosis).[5] This is important information for treating physicians.

- Concordance or discrepancy between the pretransplant diagnosis and the pathologic diagnosis of the explants provides invaluable feedback to the clinical team.

- The ventricles are almost always somewhat dilated, even in the absence of any clinical signs or symptoms. Similarly the ventricles are almost always somewhat hypertrophied.[6]

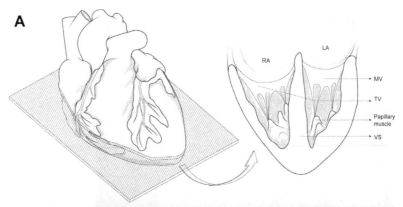

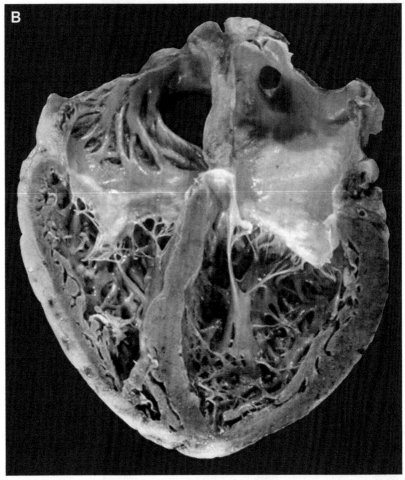

Fig. 5. (A) Schematic illustrating four chamber cut. LA, left atrium; MV, mitral valve; RA, right atrium; TV, tricuspid valve; VS, ventricular septum. *(B)* Cut section of heart showing dilated cardiomyopathy with severe atrial and ventricular dilation.

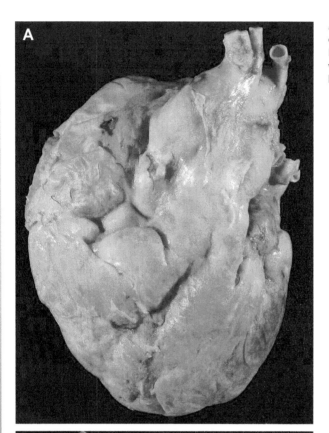

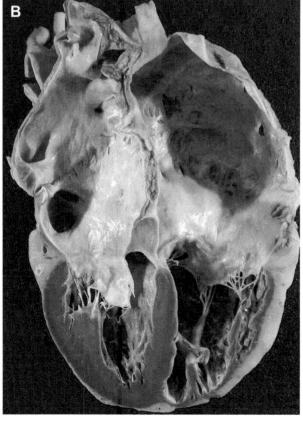

Fig. 6. (*A*) Failed allograft (from autopsy) with dense epicardial adhesions and suture lines. (*B*) Four chamber cut showing atrial suture line with "double atria" from a transplant in which biatrial anastomosis had been performed.

THE ALLOGRAFT (RE-TRANSPLANTATION)

The most common cause of allograft failure necessitating retransplantation is allograft coronary disease. Retransplantation may also be performed for hyperacute rejection in the immediate postoperative period. In some cases, intractable acute rejection has necessitated retransplantation.

Allograft coronary disease is characterized by concentric intimal proliferation of epicardial and intramyocardial vessels which results in secondary ischemic changes to the myocardium. The explanted allograft heart with allograft coronary disease should be examined using the same general technique as outlined for ischemic heart disease. Document what is included in the specimen, including the previous surgical anastomoses in the atria and great arteries. Note whether the anastomoses are well-healed and intact. Recipient atria may be included (Fig. 6), depending upon where the surgical anastomoses are made. There may be two fossae ovalis and possibly two sinoatrial nodes if the older atrial to atrial anastomosis was used. Alternatively, a four-chamber cut may be used for evaluation of rejection, chamber dimensions, and other intracavitary pathology such as fibrosis or thrombosis.

Diagnostic considerations must include allograft-related problems such as acute rejection and transplant arteriopathy with secondary changes to the myocardium. Acute rejection, when severe, may account for failure of the allograft. However, less severe rejection may be found in myocardial sections of allografts which failed from other causes. In addition, the pathologist must also take care to note underlying natural disease that may have developed or progressed in the donor heart, independent of the transplant procedure. The coronary arteries should be carefully examined as usual for the development of transplant arteriopathy or atherosclerotic disease. The myocardium should be examined for acute rejection, infarcts, drug-related changes, and hypertensive changes.[7]

SUMMARY

The dissection of an explanted heart is one of the more challenging specimens faced by the surgical pathologist for a number of reasons including relative unfamiliarity of the surgical pathologist with cardiac pathology, complexity of underlying cardiac conditions, variety and type of prior surgical procedures and importance of correctly identifying and diagnosing inheritable conditions. This was a general review of dissection techniques used for different cardiac conditions leading to transplantation. Cardiac pathology consultations are often helpful is difficult cases.

ACKNOWLEDGMENTS

The author would like to thank Drs Emily R. Duncanson and Shannon M. Mackey-Bojack of the Jesse E. Edwards Registry of Cardiovascular Disease for much useful discussion and help with this article.

REFERENCES

1. Scholz DG, Kitzman DW, Hagen PT, et al. Age-related changes in normal human hearts during the first 10 decades of life. Part I. Growth. A quantitative anatomic study of 100 specimens from subjects from birth to 19 years old. Mayo Clin Proc 1988;63:126.

2. Bradshaw SH, Kennedy L, Dexter DF, et al. A practical method to rapidly dissolve metallic stents. Cardiovasc Pathol 2009;18(3):127–33.

3. Harris KM, Spirito P, Maron MS, et al. Prevalence, clinical profile and significance of left ventricular remodeling in the end stage phase of hypertrophic cardiomyopathy. Circulation 2006;114:216–25.

4. Mackey-Bojack SM, Roe SJ, Titus JL. Sudden death with circumferential subepicardial fibrofatty replacement: left-sided arrhythmogenic ventricular cardiomyopathy. Am J Forensic Med Pathol 2009;30(2):209–14.

5. Billingham ME. Pathology of human cardiac transplantation. In: Schoen FJ, Gimbrone MA, editors. Cardiovascular pathology: clinicopathologic correlations and pathogenetic mechanisms. Baltimore (MD): Williams & Wilkins; 1995. p. 108.

6. Rowan RA, Billingham ME. Pathologic changes in the long-term transplanted heart: a morphometric study of myocardial hypertrophy, vascularity and fibrosis. Hum Pathol 1990;21:767.

7. McManus BM, Markin RS. The role of the autopsy in transplantation. In: Kolbeck PC, Markin RS, editors. Transplant pathology. Chicago: American Society of Clinical Pathologists; 1994. p. 311–4.

PATHOLOGIC EVALUATION OF CARDIOVASCULAR MEDICAL DEVICES

Robert F. Padera, MD, PhD

KEYWORDS

• Medical device • Complications • Stent • Ventricular assist device • Cardiovascular • Pathology

ABSTRACT

Cardiovascular devices such as coronary artery stents, ventricular assist devices, pacemakers, automated implantable cardioverter-defibrillators and septal closure devices are life saving and improve quality of life for millions of patients each year. Complications of these devices include thrombosis/thromboembolism, infection, structural failure and adverse material-tissue interactions. These findings should be sought when these devices are encountered on the surgical pathology bench or at autopsy.

INTRODUCTION

Cardiac surgeons and interventional cardiologists have been leaving their calling cards in the cardiovascular system for almost 60 and 30 years, respectively, and the evaluation of their handiwork has been the province of the cardiovascular pathologist ever since. These interventions and devices have contributed to increased longevity and improved quality of life for countless individuals, and represent some of the greatest successes of modern medicine. Because of their increasing use in the industrialized world, cardiovascular devices such as coronary artery stents, prosthetic heart valves, septal closure devices, ventricular assist devices, pacemakers and automated implanted cardioverter-defibrillators are encountered with increasing frequency by pathologists both on the surgical pathology bench and in the autopsy suite. Proper pathologic evaluation of these devices is important for patient care, but also for identifying mechanisms of failure (or impending failure) of these devices to inform designs of the next generation of implants and to mitigate risk for other patients with the same devices still in place. The inefficiency of postmarketing surveillance of implanted medical devices is an ongoing problem that is currently building to a crescendo[1–3]; having reliable pathologic data is one critical component of correcting this issue.

A handful of predictable pathogenic pathways underlie the eventual degeneration or failure of these various interventions in most cases; occasionally an untoward and unexpected complication can be the culprit.[4] For any device in the cardiovascular system, thrombosis and thromboembolism are major considerations. The risk of thrombosis is increased in the absence of intact, functional endothelium in contact with blood, as is the case for most of the devices discussed here. Anticoagulation with medications such as antiplatelet agents, warfarin, heparin and other novel therapeutics required to prevent thrombosis of some cardiovascular devices increases bleeding risk, and may lead to subsequent fatal hemorrhage elsewhere. The risk of infection is increased in the presence of a foreign body largely due to the ability of certain organisms to form protective biofilm. For devices that have ongoing continuity with the outside world such as ventricular assist devices via the driveline, infection becomes a major source of morbidity and mortality. Material-tissue interactions, including exuberant or defective healing, chronic inflammation and even hypersensitivity reactions, can lead to dysfunction of implantable devices. For coronary artery stents, the problem of restenosis falls into this category. Structural

Department of Pathology, Brigham and Women's Hospital, 75 Francis Street, Boston, MA 02115, USA
E-mail address: rpadera@partners.org

Surgical Pathology 5 (2012) 497–521
doi:10.1016/j.path.2012.04.001
1875-9181/12/$ – see front matter © 2012 Published by Elsevier Inc.

degeneration, such as calcification of bioprosthetic heart valves, fractures of metallic device components in stented devices or wear of moving parts in ventricular assist devices, is always an issue in inert materials or in tissue that cannot repair itself.

This article focuses on coronary artery stents, ventricular assist devices, implantable cardioverter-defibrillators and septal closure devices. It highlights typical failure modes, and presents approaches to evaluate these devices on the surgical pathology bench. Along with prosthetic heart valves (VanderLaan, Padera, Schoen: *Practical approach to evaluation of prosthetic heart valves* in this publication), these represent both the most commonly encountered devices, as well as those where dysfunction most commonly contributes to morbidity and mortality.

CORONARY ARTERY STENTS

Stents are expandable tubes of metallic mesh that splint open the coronary artery at the site of balloon angioplasty to preserve luminal patency and minimize thrombus formation.[5,6] They have been used in the treatment of atherosclerotic coronary artery and ischemic heart disease for over three decades, and stand as one of the major success stories in engineering and medicine.[7] Stenting may involve any part of the coronary arteries or saphenous vein grafts, distal to proximal, and even extend across branch points. Currently used devices are classified as either bare-metal stents or drug-eluting stents. Most drug-eluting stents are composed of a metal stent with a polymer coating that releases a medication (paclitaxel, sirolimus or similar drug) that minimizes the intimal proliferation that causes restenosis.[8-10] Although the differences between bare metal stents and drug-eluting stents are not apparent grossly or radiologically, they have different short- and long-term risks of thrombosis and restenosis.[11] Stents that are entirely bioresorbable, leaving behind no foreign material after they fully degrade, are under development and in clinical trials.[12,13]

The pathologist will encounter stents on the surgical pathology bench in explanted hearts, most often in patients whose indication for transplantation was atherosclerotic coronary artery and ischemic heart disease. Acute changes in the stents such as fresh thrombosis are unusual in this setting, as patients are rarely transplanted in the middle of an acute event. In the autopsy suite, however, acute stent thrombosis occurring either early or late after implantation may indeed represent the cause of death.

Key Points
STENTS

- Dissect the coronary arteries from the heart and perform a radiograph to identify stents
- Avoid opening or disrupting the stents; either special resin embedding with subsequent sectioning should be performed, or the stent should be electrochemically dissolved before processing
- Restenosis via intimal hyperplasia is a common pathology with bare metal stents; drug eluting stents are designed to minimize this problem
- Occlusive thrombus can occur early or late after implantation; drug eluting stents have a higher incidence of late stent thrombosis than bare metal stents

Gross Evaluation

The clinical history of the patient should be ascertained, as catheterization or operative reports can be helpful in determining number, location and configuration of any stents that have been placed as well as any associated technical or clinical issues. After taking gross photographs of the explanted heart, the coronary arteries should be carefully dissected from the heart (Fig. 1A), minimizing handling that can introduce artifactual stent deformation. Serial transverse sections of the heart can then be performed to characterize the nature and extent of the ischemic heart disease. Gross palpation for stents is insufficiently sensitive to localize the stents, and is further confounded by the presence of calcified arterial lesions. After fixation, the coronaries should be placed in a decalcification solution; this does not affect the ability to process or evaluate the stented segments. Either before or after decalcification, the coronaries should be radiographed to identify the areas of stent placement (Fig. 1B), the adequacy of deployment and the presence of damage or fractures of the stent.[14] The non-stented portions of the arteries should be thinly sectioned (Fig. 2) to ascertain the extent and location of atherosclerotic lesions and to evaluate the vessel for procedure-related pathologies such as dissection that can occur with instrumentation. The intact stented sections can be grossly inspected to determine patency by looking down the lumen (as one would use a telescope) before further evaluation.

The stented segments of artery require unique processing; if they are not removed from the heart

Fig. 1. Coronary dissection and radiography. (*A*) The coronary arteries should be dissected from the heart as intact segments. The arteries including segments containing stents can be fixed in formalin and decalcified. (*B*) Areas of stent deployment (*arrows*) can be identified on a specimen radiograph.

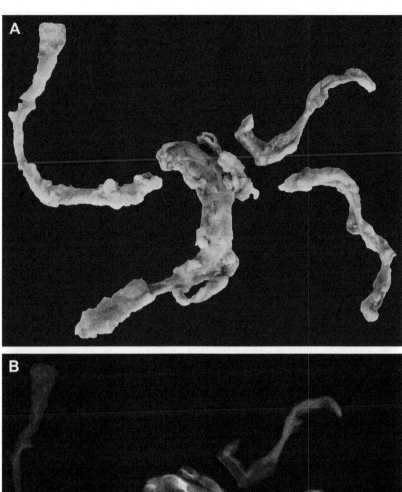

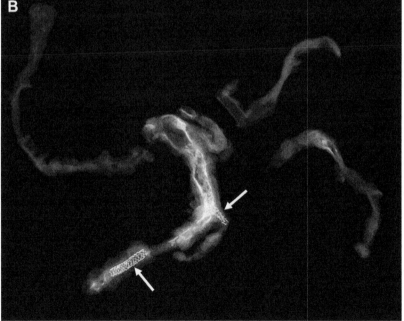

and specifically preserved, the opportunity for any reliable assessment of their patency will be lost. The entire segment of the vessel that is stented should be preserved intact, and intact stents should never be removed from the stented vessel which would completely disrupt any pathology that may be present. While some reports suggest that the stents can be opened longitudinally with scissors,[15] this is not preferred in our experience. Some groups report success removing stent struts after cutting them axially with diamond scissors.[16] Attempts to remove intact stents will only disrupt

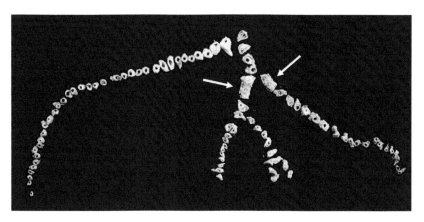

Fig. 2. Coronary dissection with stented segments. After identifying the stented areas on the radiograph, the remainder of the coronary vasculature can be serially sectioned to assess degree of stenosis and any acute plaque changes while leaving the stented segments intact (*arrows*).

the vessel and destroy any pathology, and should be avoided.

Microscopic Evaluation

The traditional method for sectioning stents involves embedding in a resin such as methylmethacrylate, sectioning with a tungsten carbide or diamond knife, with additional microgrinding to achieve a thin section that can then be stained, as might be done for non-decalcified bone.[17,18] As these capabilities are not available in many centers, stented segments of vessels can be submitted to one of a handful of national laboratories that will embed and produce sections at intervals along the vessel. This approach requires more time and specimen handling, plus may incur a financial cost. However, the histology is superior. Two such facilities are CVPath Institute, Inc. (Gaithersburg, MD, USA), and CBSET, Inc., (Lexington, MA, USA). A novel processing method that is amenable to set up in any lab involves electrochemically dissolving the stents by a process akin to electroplating, followed by routine histologic processing.[19] Using a power source and other routinely available equipment, a stented vessel can usually be sectioned after less than a day. Locations of thromboses and intimal hyperplasia are not affected by the treatment, and acute lesions associated with cause of death in the autopsy setting can be reliably identified. Routine H&E staining should be performed; trichrome and elastin staining may be useful in determining the extent of intimal proliferation and presence of dissection or other pathologies.

Pathology of Coronary Artery Stents

Stented vessel segments may occlude because of thrombosis which may happen soon after stent deployment or much later (so-called late stent thrombosis), or due to chronic concentric intimal hyperplasia leading to restenosis.

In the setting of a stent, thrombosis (**Fig. 3**) generally occurs because of endothelial injury, with the risk being the greatest until the stent and underlying vessel have been re-endothelialized. The risk of stent thrombosis in the immediate post-procedure interval is greatly diminished by current anticoagulant pharmacotherapy. A small amount of platelet-fibrin thrombus coating the struts is likely always present in the days after stenting, but this typically wanes after about a month. However, late stent thrombosis has become a concern, especially with drug-eluting stents.[20] It is thought that drug-eluting stents demonstrate delayed arterial healing accompanied by poor endothelialization of stent struts[21]; this provides the nidus for thrombosis, especially after potent antiplatelet agents are discontinued. Such endothelialization is also slowed by disrupted, bent, fractured, or overlapping stents.[22]

Long-term, stents may undergo concentric intimal hyperplasia that can be flow-limiting and a cause of ischemia.[23] Bare metal stents tend to develop such concentric stenoses at a faster rate, leading to potentially significant occlusion in 50% within 5 years (**Fig. 4**). Drug-eluting stents have a better long-term profile with significant stenosis in only 20 to 30% of patients after the same interval (**Fig. 5**). Intimal proliferation consists of smooth muscle-like cells within extracellular matrix that can range from loose to dense (**Fig. 6**). A foreign body giant cell reaction adjacent to the elements of the stent (**Fig. 7**) can be seen with associated mild chronic inflammation including a predominance of macrophages.[24] Eosinophils may also be present, suggesting a hypersensitivity component to some element of the stent or polymer matrix

Fig. 3. Drug eluting stent with thrombosis. Whole mount section showing stent with chronic, partially recanalized thrombosis. The stent struts can be identified as the empty geometric shapes (*arrows*). Hematoxylin and eosin stain.

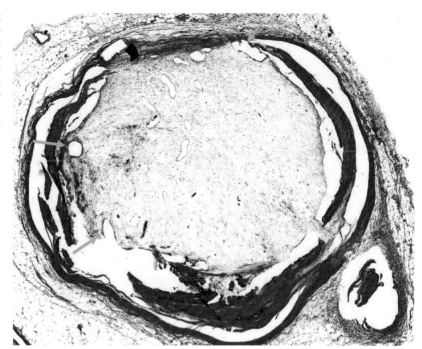

Fig. 4. Bare metal stent with restenosis after 2 years. Whole mount section showing moderate intimal proliferation which significantly narrows the lumen. The outlines of the stent struts (*arrows*) mark the diameter of the lumen immediately after stenting. Hematoxylin and eosin stain.

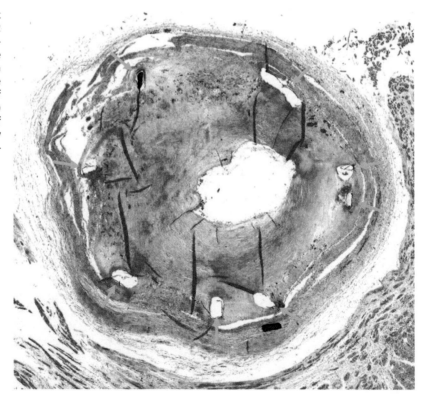

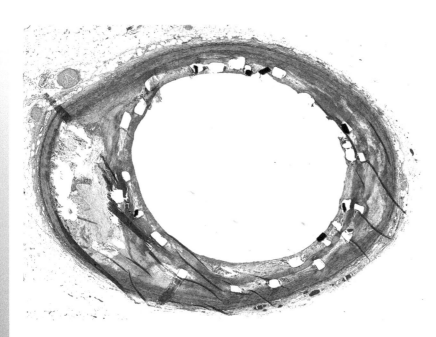

Fig. 5. Drug eluting stent with minimal restenosis after 3 years. Whole mount section showing minimal intimal proliferation and maintenance of the luminal cross-sectional area. This section is taken from an area of two overlapping stents, hence the concentric ringed appearance of the stent struts. Hematoxylin and eosin stain.

of drug-eluting stents. The polymer matrix of drug-eluting stents may occasionally be seen as a thin basophilic amorphous coating on the metallic elements. Embolic material is occasionally seen downstream in the coronary microvasculature distal to these stents (**Fig. 8**), which may represent the polymer matrix of the stent or polymers from the catheters used to deploy them.[25]

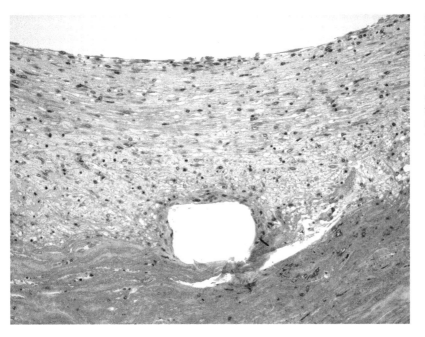

Fig. 6. Intimal proliferation. Photomicrograph showing moderate intimal proliferation consisting of smooth muscle-like spindle cells in a loose collagen matrix with a sparse chronic inflammatory infiltrate. Hematoxylin and eosin stained section, 10× objective.

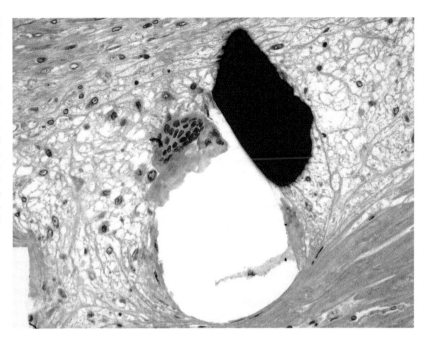

Fig. 7. Foreign body giant cell reaction. Photomicrograph showing foreign body giant cells adjacent to the stent strut with surrounding loose connective tissue containing smooth muscle-like cells, macrophages and occasional lymphocytes. The metallic strut has been slightly pushed through the tissue during sectioning, accounting for the apparent artifact. Hematoxylin and eosin stained section, 20× objective.

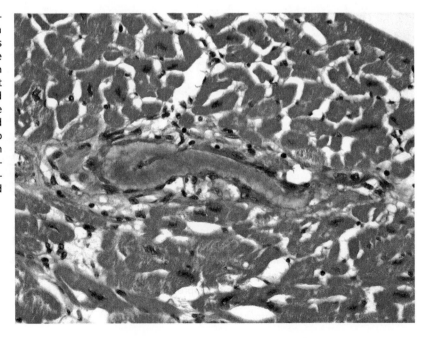

Fig. 8. Polymer microembolus. Photomicrograph showing a microembolus of polymer within the myocardium either from the drug-eluting stent matrix or catheter used to deploy the stent. The polymer is basophilic and has started to develop an inflammatory reaction around it within the occluded small vessel. Hematoxylin and eosin stained section, 20× objective.

VENTRICULAR ASSIST DEVICES

Mechanical circulatory support,[26] such as a ventricular assist device (VAD) or a total artificial heart, is generally used in two main settings. Patients can receive a device as a "bridge to transplantation" for those eligible for a heart transplant,[27] or as "destination therapy" for those with heart failure who are ineligible for transplantation for whatever reason.[28,29] Rarely, patients may recover their native cardiac function after a period of VAD support enough to allow removal of the device; "bridge to recovery" is the term used for this indication.[30] Pathologists may therefore receive these devices on the surgical bench when they are explanted:

1. At the time of heart transplantation
2. At the time of device replacement for device malfunction
3. At the time of recovery of native cardiac function when the device is no longer required.

A wide variety of cardiac assist and replacement devices are in preclinical development, in clinical trials, and in routine use around the world.[31] These include implantable pulsatile devices such as the Thoratec HeartMate XVE (**Fig. 9**) and the Thoratec IVAD (**Fig. 10**), paracorporeal pulsatile devices such as the Thoratec PVAD (**Fig. 11**) and the Berlin Heart EXCOR, implantable continuous flow devices such as the DeBakey VAD, the Jarvik 2000, and the Thoratec HeartMate II (**Fig. 12**), percutaneous continuous flow devices[32,33] such as the CardiacAssist TandemHeart (**Fig. 13**) and the Abiomed Impella Recover, and total artificial hearts such as the SynCardia (CardioWest) Total Artificial Heart (**Fig. 14**)[34] and the Abiomed Abio-Cor Implantable Replacement Heart. The first step in evaluation of a ventricular assist device is

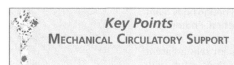

> **Key Points**
> MECHANICAL CIRCULATORY SUPPORT
>
> - Mechanical circulatory support can be used as a bridge to transplantation or as the permanent solution for patients with end-stage heart failure.
>
> - An explanted heart can be dissected as it would be if no device were present; the device should be disassembled to the extent possible to evaluate for pathologic findings.
>
> - Thrombosis (either in the device or native heart), infection, changes in the native heart, structural device problems, and adverse device-patient interactions are the most common pathologic findings; often the device is unremarkable in a patient successfully bridged to transplantation.

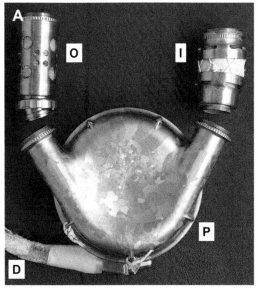

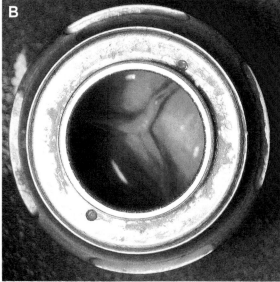

Fig. 9. Thoratec HeartMate XVE. (*A*) Gross photograph showing inflow conduit (I), pump (P), outflow conduit (O) and driveline (D). (*B*) Gross photograph of bioprosthetic porcine aortic valve that serves as the inflow valve for this pulsatile pump. A similar valve is present in the outflow conduit. The inflow valve in particular would suffer structural failure manifest as cuspal tears.

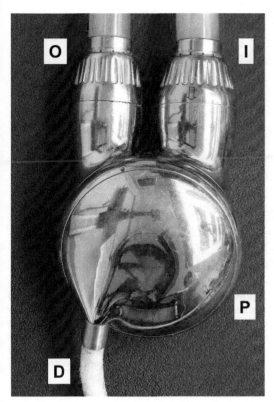

Fig. 10. Thoratec IVAD. Gross photograph showing inflow conduit (I), pump (P), outflow conduit (O) and driveline (D) for this implanted pulsatile pump with mechanical valves on the inflow and outflow aspects.

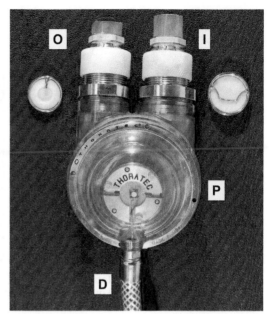

Fig. 11. Thoratec PVAD. Gross photograph showing inflow conduit (I), pump (P), outflow conduit (O) and driveline (D) for this paracorporeal pulsatile pump with mechanical valves on the inflow and outflow aspects. The valves are shown separately from the conduits in this photo.

to identify the device type. At our institution and in the US at the time of this writing, the most commonly explanted devices are shown in **Figs. 9–14**, with the HeartMate II being the most

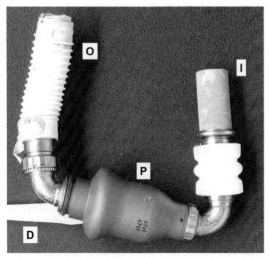

Fig. 12. Thoratec HeartMate II. Gross photograph showing inflow conduit (I), pump (P), outflow conduit (O) and proximal portion of the driveline (D) for this implanted continuous flow axial pump.

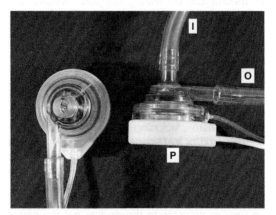

Fig. 13. CardiacAssist Tandem Heart. Gross photograph showing top and side views of this paracorporeal percutaneous continuous flow centrifugal pump. The inflow (I) to the pump (P) is connected to a long cannula that is inserted into the femoral vein, directed into the right atrium and across the interatrial septum via septal puncture to rest in the left atrium; the outflow (O) is inserted into the femoral artery. The magnetically-driven impeller is best seen (*arrow*) from the top view.

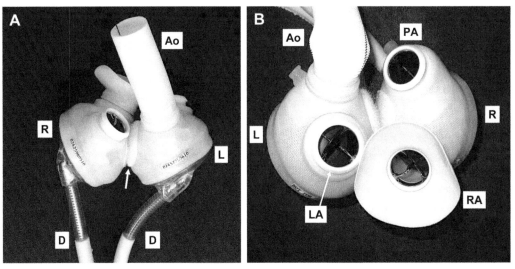

Fig. 14. Syncardia (CardioWest) Total Artificial Heart. (*A*) Gross photograph from the anterior aspect of the device showing the left (L) and right (R) pumps. The Dacron graft represents the outflow from the left pump and would be anastomosed to the native ascending aorta (Ao). There is Velcro holding the right and left pumps together (*arrow*), allowing for optimal positioning to conform to the patient's anatomy at implantation. The drivelines (D) are also seen. (*B*) Gross photograph of from the superior-posterior aspect of the device. The anastomosis to the native pulmonary artery (PA) is also made via a Dacron graft (not shown). The area of anastomosis to the native right atrium (RA) and left atrium (LA) are as indicated. All of the device valves are Medtronic-Hall type mechanical valves.

common. This section is not meant to provide an exhaustive description of all of these devices, but rather to highlight an approach to the evaluation of mechanical circulatory support devices and illustrate various pathologic findings related to their use.

Gross Evaluation

As is true in most areas of pathology, understanding the clinical history is an important part of the device evaluation. Communication with the clinical team including cardiologist, cardiac surgeon and/or VAD coordinator can be useful in determining the indication for explant, as well as whether the device needs to be returned to the manufacturer after pathologic examination.

The convention is to name the cannulae based on their relationship to the device, not the native heart; thus, the inflow cannula directs blood from the heart into the VAD while the outflow conduit directs blood out of the VAD and into the circulation. Left ventricular assist devices (Fig. 15) generally consist of:

1. Inflow cannula that exits the left ventricular chamber through the apex of the heart

2. Axial flow or centrifugal pump which may sit in the peritoneal cavity, in a pre-peritoneal pocket, or in the pericardial space
3. Outflow cannula and graft which anastomose to the ascending aorta
4. Driveline attached to the pump itself that is tunneled in the subcutaneous tissue to exit through the skin to the right of the abdominal midline
5. External hardware such as a controller and batteries.

Right ventricular assist devices usually have the inflow cannula placed in the right atrium due to the small size and unfavorable geometry of the right ventricle with the outflow graft anastomosed to the main pulmonary artery. Total artificial hearts will be orthotopic and completely replace the native ventricles.

A systematic approach to the evaluation of these devices will serve the pathologist well and will allow documentation of the pertinent findings. One approach for devices received with an explanted heart is to:

1. Evaluate the driveline with any attached soft tissue.

Fig. 15. Thoratec Heart-Mate II with heart. Gross photograph showing the inflow cannula (I) inserted into the left ventricle, the pump (P), driveline (D) and outflow (O) cannula and graft anastomosed to the ascending aorta.

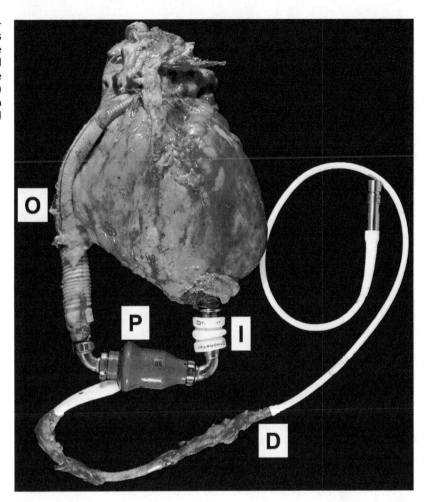

2. Evaluate the attachments of the device to the native heart at the left ventricular apex and ascending aorta.
3. Open the heart to demonstrate the appropriate native cardiac pathology (eg, transverse sections for ischemic heart disease [Fig. 16], 4-chamber cut for dilated cardiomyopathy [Fig. 17]).
4. Partially disassemble the device into component parts and evaluate for intra-device pathology along the lines of flow through the device.
5. Evaluate the native heart and any other received tissues for signs of pathologies induced by the ventricular assist device.

Devices received as separate specimens can be disassembled and evaluated along the lines of flow.

Devices, along with the native heart, should be photographed to document the device type and the tissue received. Requests for the return of the device to the manufacturer may occur to allow for evaluation of various additional structural and functional components, and these requests should be accommodated if possible after pathologic evaluation.

Microscopic Evaluation

Microscopic sections of tissue adherent to the driveline or any aspect of the device are warranted in cases of suspected infection. Areas of anastomotic dehiscence should also be sectioned to determine the viability of adjacent tissues and to rule out infection.

Pathology of Ventricular Assist Devices

The most common pathologic findings associated with mechanical circulatory support include thrombosis and thromboembolism, hemorrhage,

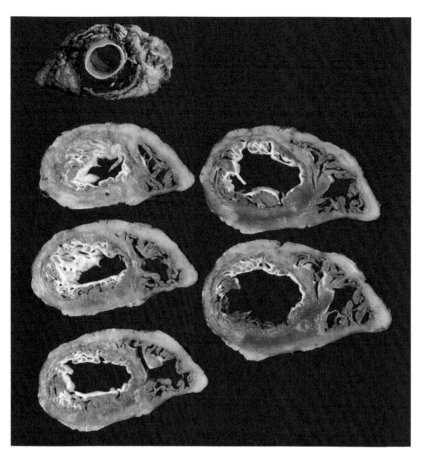

Fig. 16. Transverse sections of ischemic heart with VAD. Gross photograph showing heart as it would be sectioned for a patient transplanted for ischemic heart disease. The inflow cannula has been removed from the apex (top photo), and transverse sections have been taken of the heart to demonstrate a remote anterior myocardial infarction.

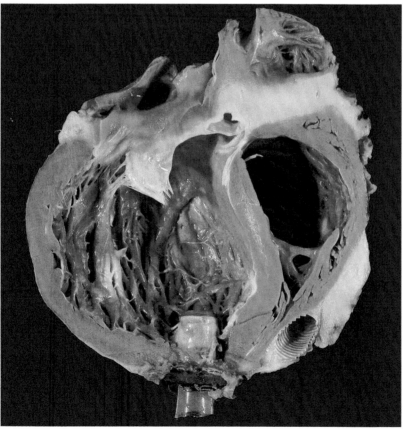

Fig. 17. Four-chamber section of DCM heart with VAD. Gross photograph showing heart as it would be sectioned for a patient transplanted for dilated cardiomyopathy. A four-chamber cut has been performed to show the ventricular dilation and position of the inflow cannula in the left ventricle from this patient with a Thoratec PVAD.

infection, changes in the native heart, structural device problems, and adverse device-patient interactions; these are the findings to seek out when evaluating these specimens.[35] However, there indeed may be no pathologic findings in the VAD of a patient who has been successfully bridged to transplantation with a clinically well-functioning device.

The soft tissue around the driveline and pump should be scrutinized for signs of necrosis, hemorrhage or abscess formation, as the driveline is a common route of device infection (Fig. 18).[36] Cultures and/or histologic sections should be taken to document infection and identify the offending organism.[37] The portion of the driveline external to the patient should be investigated for signs of wear, erosion or mechanical damage.

The location of the inflow cannula within the left ventricular chamber should be noted along with any possible impingement on native heart structures or evidence of dehiscence from the insertion site leading to hemorrhage. The inflow cannula should be evaluated for thrombosis, vegetations, structural or anastomotic failure, and pannus formation. For most pumps, the inflow and outflow cannulas can generally be detached from the pump to allow better visualization of the device lumen by unscrewing the connectors. The pump itself generally should not be opened, but one can visualize most of the pumping chamber using a properly-oriented bright light. The pump should be evaluated primarily for the presence of thrombus (Figs. 19 and 20) or vegetations. The serial number of the pump should be noted. Similar to the inflow cannula, the outflow cannula should be evaluated for thrombosis (Fig. 21), vegetations, kinking, structural failure, and anastomotic failure.

Evaluation of the native heart is important because the presence of the VAD can induce important changes. The aortic valve may only infrequently open during mechanical circulatory support because blood is pumped from the left ventricular chamber to the ascending aorta effectively bypassing the aortic valve. Over time, the cusps may partially or completely fuse (Fig. 22) leading to stenosis (which is inconsequential as long as the device is working), insufficiency, or thrombus formation.[38] Just as thrombi are predisposed to form in areas of disturbed flow inside the device, they can also form in the native heart where the presence of the device may lead to abnormal flow patterns. These thrombi (Fig. 23) can form in areas adjacent to the inflow cannula or on the ventricular surface of the aortic valve as mentioned above,

and can be the source of thromboembolic complications. A heart supported by a VAD for a prolonged period of time can undergo reverse remodeling; that is, the left ventricular chamber will return toward a normal size from its original dilated state. Thus, at the time of transplantation, the inflow cannula in the left ventricular apex may contact areas of the now-smaller heart that it was not interacting with when the device was implanted (Fig. 24). This can lead to obstruction to flow to the VAD and circulatory compromise. If the inflow cannula significantly impinges on the interventricular septum, it can erode through the muscular wall resulting in a ventricular septal defect.

PACEMAKERS AND AUTOMATED IMPLANTABLE CARDIOVERTER-DEFIBRILLATORS

Pacemakers are implanted to maintain a minimum or fixed heart rate, or to better synchronize biventricular contraction for patients with congestive heart failure. Implantable cardioverter-defibrillators (ICD) are implanted to cardiovert patients who develop life-threatening arrhythmias. Many devices have both pacing and defibrillating capabilities.[39,40] These devices are typically implanted as subcutaneous units containing the control circuitry and power supply connected to leads that run via a subclavian vein and superior vena cava into the right heart. Pacers most commonly have dual leads implanted into both the right atrium and right ventricle (and the coronary sinus to access the left ventricle for biventricular pacing), whereas ICDs only have a single lead in the right ventricular apex.

These devices interact with a variety of host tissues, including the subcutaneous pocket where the body of the device sits, the venous walls, the right atrial walls, the tricuspid valve, the right ventricle and possibly the coronary sinus. Within the subcutaneous tissue, a bland fibrous capsule usually forms around the device as would be predicted for a large foreign body. The leads within the veins and right atrium often become ensheathed within a fibrous capsule that may anchor the leads to the vein or atrial wall. The leads cross the tricuspid valve and engender variable degrees of tricuspid valve scarring and associated regurgitation; however, these are usually not clinically significant as the valve can usually close around the lead (like lips around a straw), even with significant entanglement of a lead with chordae or leaflets. The ends of the leads are designed for optimal interaction with host tissue, to provide anchoring

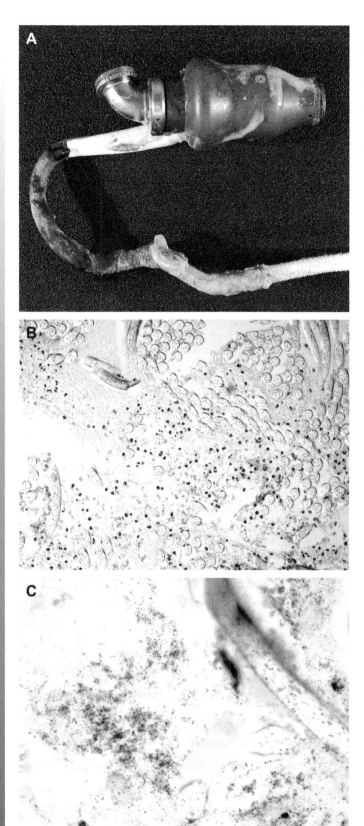

Fig. 18. Infection. (*A*) Gross photograph of pump and driveline with frank pus and necrotic debris on the device components. (*B*) Photomicrograph of driveline showing no significant tissue ingrowth or healing, but with acute inflammation. Hematoxylin and eosin stained section, 10× objective. (*C*) Photomicrograph of driveline showing innumerable bacteria within the interstices of the driveline. Gram stain, 40× objective.

Fig. 19. Thrombosis of TandemHeart. (*A*) Gross photograph of inflow cannula that had been present in the left atrium with large thrombus on the tip. (*B*) Gross photograph of pump with thrombosis within the pumping chamber from the same patient.

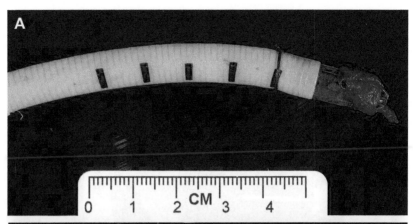

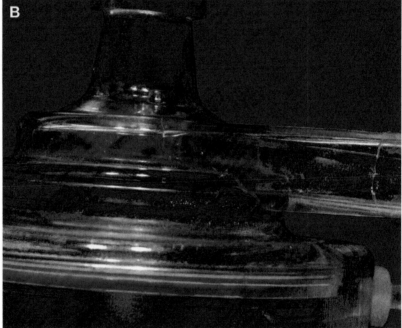

and close contact with the myocardium while minimizing the fibrous reaction.

Pathologist Evaluation of Pacemakers and Implantable Cardioverter-Defibrillators

Surgical pathologists will encounter pacemakers and ICDs either within explanted hearts or as separately submitted specimens. Evaluation of the devices and attached tissue is important to document the indication for removal and to correlate device complications with the clinical trajectory of the patient. For all devices, the make, model and serial number should be recorded and gross photographs taken to document the devices and relevant findings. The number and configuration of the leads should be described as well as any attached soft tissue. If pacer or ICD dysfunction is a consideration

for a sudden death in the autopsy setting, the device should be interrogated by the electrophysiology service; this may provide important information about potential terminal rhythms and activity of the pacer/ICD before death and can establish whether the device was functioning properly.

Pathology of Pacemakers and Implantable Cardioverter-Defibrillators

Pacemakers and ICDs share many of the same complications, often requiring device removal and replacement. Like many cardiovascular devices, these are life sustaining technologies and the implications of device failure can be fatal due to a lack of appropriate cardiac pacing (for pacemakers) or inability to sense or deliver appropriate therapy for a lethal arrhythmia (for ICDs). While normal

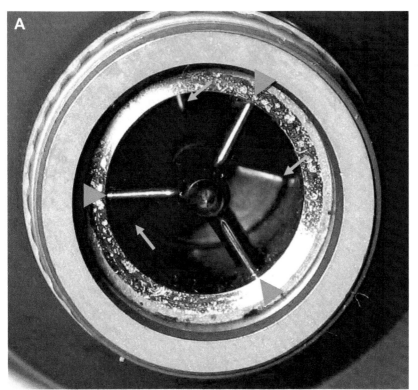

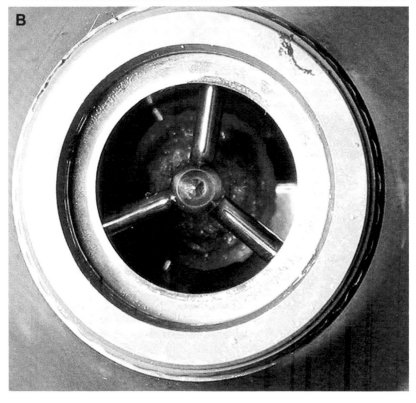

Fig. 20. Thrombosis of HeartMate II. (*A*) Gross photograph of inflow aspect of a normal HeartMate II after disconnecting the inflow cannula and housing. The outer three spokes (*arrowheads*) represent the flow straightener, while the impeller is visible (*arrows*) deep to the flow straightener. (*B*) Gross photograph of large thrombus at the bearing between the impeller and flow straightener on the inflow aspect of the pump.

Fig. 21. Outflow anastomotic thrombosis. Gross photograph of anastomosis between outflow cannula and ascending aorta. There is mild pannus overgrowth at the anastomosis along with an organizing thrombus (*arrow*).

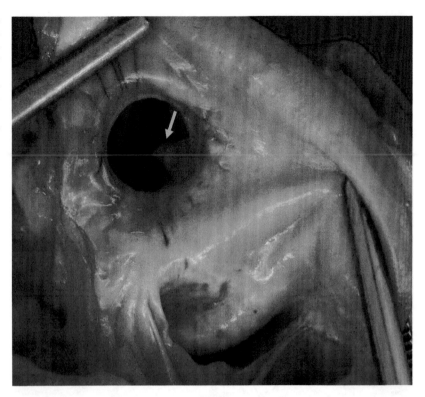

device end-of-service from a depleted battery may not be technically considered a device malfunction, it certainly requires device replacement, and may happen prematurely due to increased fibrosis at the lead-tissue interface requiring a higher stimulus threshold. Failures of the hardware, including the battery/capacitor and charge circuit, connectors and leads are the most common device malfunctions, with software problems being less prevalent. Some mechanical failures include electrode

Fig. 22. Cuspal fusion. Gross photograph of the native aortic valve opened through the non-coronary cusp in a patient after a long period of support with HeartMate XVE. The right and left coronary cusps (*arrows*) are fused together from commissure to coaptation point.

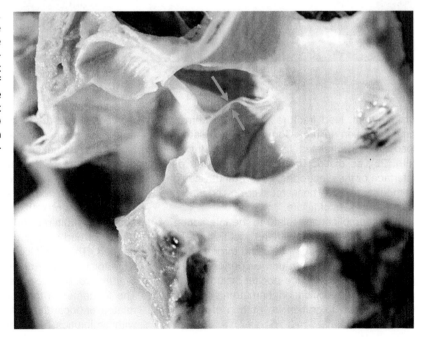

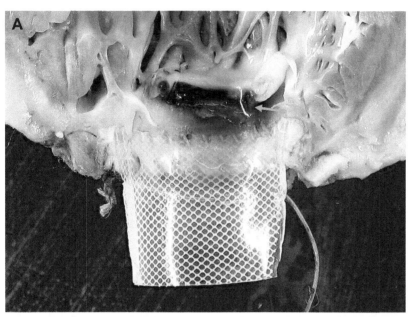

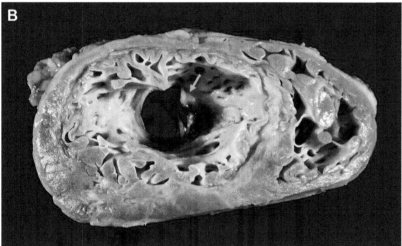

Fig. 23. Thrombi within heart. (A) Gross photograph showing organizing thrombus (arrow) at the junction of the inflow cannula and left ventricle in a patient supported with a HeartMate II. The pre-transplant course of the patient was characterized by transient ischemic attacks. (B) Gross photograph showing organizing thrombus (arrow) at the junction of the inflow cannula and left ventricle in a patient supported with a HeartMate XVE.

dislodgment, lead fractures, electrode corrosion and insulation failure. Complications related to leads may be related to the body of the lead (Fig. 25), as distinct from the lead-device pack interface or the electrodes.[41] Several devices and components have been recalled in recent years for these modes of failure.[42]

Many complications relate to the interaction of the device biomaterials with the host tissue. These include: infection; thrombosis and thromboembolism; myocardial penetration or perforation; and pathologies of the device pocket including, pressure necrosis, calcification, hematoma or seroma formation, and migration or rotation of the body of the device.

Infection is a dreaded complication of implantable devices in general, and is this is certainly true for pacemakers and ICDs.[43] The infection may originate in the subcutaneous pocket and track along the lead, which acts as a contaminated foreign body. If portions of the pocket or adherent tissues are sent with the device and infection is suspected, cultures and histologic sections should be performed with appropriate special stains as needed. The most common organisms responsible for these infections are coagulase-negative Staphylococcus species such as S epidermidis. The fundamental therapeutic principle in device-related endocarditis is treatment of the infection with antibiotics followed by removal of at least

Fig. 24. Impingement. Gross photograph showing inflow cannula from a Thoratec PVAD in the left ventricular apex, the tip of which is partially buried in the interventricular septum (*arrow*). The pre-transplant course was characterized by poor VAD flows secondary to inflow obstruction.

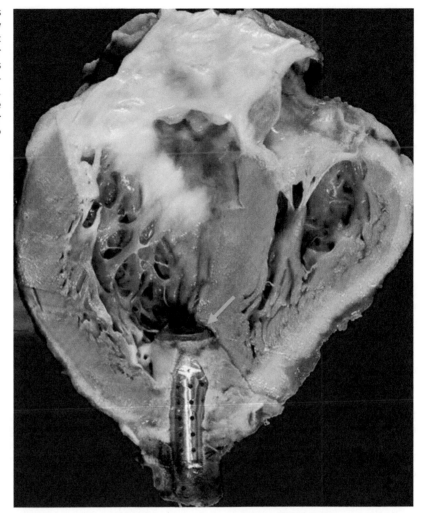

Fig. 25. Lead body erosion. Gross photograph showing a portion of a St. Jude Riata lead where the thin insulated conducting cable (*blue*) has eroded through the silicone housing to become externalized.

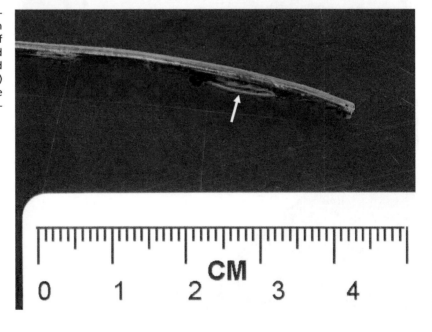

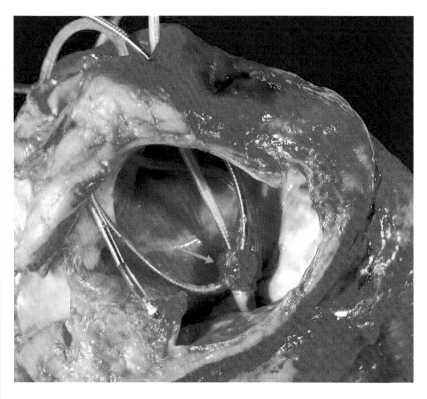

Fig. 26. Lead thrombosis. Gross photograph of the partially opened right atrium showing a recent thrombus (*arrow*) at the junction of the straight right ventricular lead and looping right atrial lead in a patient with a pacemaker.

the lead and, when the pacemaker pocket is involved, the entire pacing system.[44] Thrombosis of the leads can occur, especially in hypercoagulable patients, and may be a source of pulmonary emboli (Fig. 26). The interaction between the leads and the myocardium should be investigated in explanted hearts, including evaluation of the degree of fibrosis around the electrode and the location of the lead within the myocardium (Fig. 27). Rarely, lead implantation can result in an acute

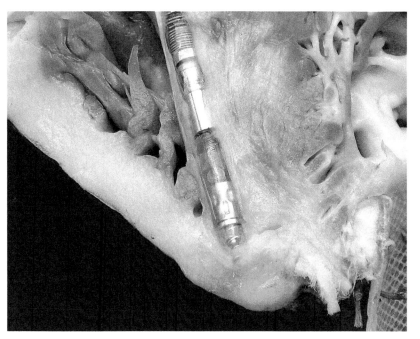

Fig. 27. Electrode position. Gross photograph showing an ICD electrode tip present in the epicardial adipose tissue rather than the myocardium with an associated fibrous reaction.

perforation. Occasionally, inflammation associated with a lead or increased pressure on the lead can cause late wall erosion. The low pressure of the right ventricle and the relatively greater pliability of the right ventricular wall generally prevents any significant pericardial bleeding or tamponade. The development of a thick pannus of fibrous tissue may be so extensive as to preclude effective signal transmission and capture, even if all other components of the device are functioning normally (**Fig. 28**). Repeated ICD discharges may lead to cycles of necrosis,

inflammation and healing which can cause fibrosis and/or ventricular wall erosion.

OCCLUSION DEVICES FOR ATRIAL OR VENTRICULAR SEPTAL DEFECTS

Atrial septal defects (ASD), including patent foramen ovale, are congenital conditions that allow flow across the interatrial septum. Ventricular septal defects (VSD) are usually congenital but can be acquired, and allow flow across the interventricular septum in a left to right direction. The

Fig. 28. Fibrous reaction to electrode tip. (*A*) Gross photograph showing minimal fibrosis at the site of insertion into the right ventricular apical myocardium. (*B*) Gross photograph showing significant fibrosis with resultant loss of capture at the site of insertion into the right ventricular apical myocardium.

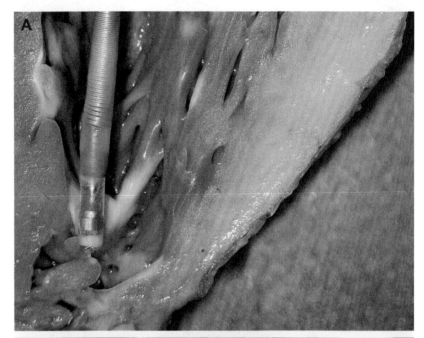

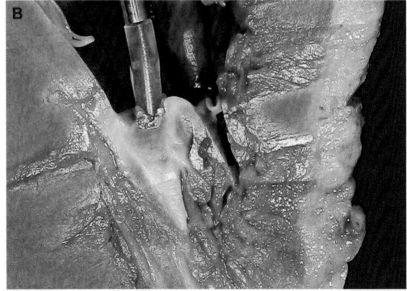

decision to close an ASD or VSD depends on the size of the defect and the symptoms of the patient. While these defects can be closed by open surgical techniques in which synthetic or bioprosthetic material is sutured over the defect, most ASDs and some VSDs can be closed via transcatheter deployment of devices which occlude the defect and allow for tissue overgrowth and healing.[45]

The Amplatzer device consists of double Nitinol discs filled with polyester patches connected by a small waist; the waist sits within the defect to connect the discs, which sit on either side of and are selected to be larger than the defect (Fig. 29). The StarFLEX device is a double umbrella device with metallic arms covered in polyester fabric; the two umbrellas are connected centrally

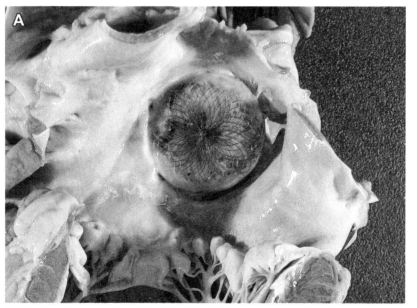

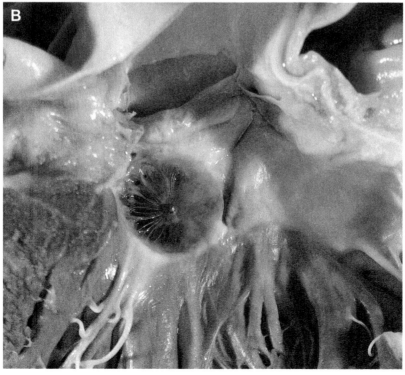

Fig. 29. Amplatzer closure devices. (A) Gross photograph of the left atrial aspect of an Amplatzer closure device deployed to close an atrial septal defect. Note the pannus overgrowth of the peripheral aspect of the wires. (B) Gross photograph of the left ventricular aspect of an Amplatzer closure device deployed to close a membranous ventricular septal defect. The metallic elements have been largely covered by thin fibrous pannus.

(Fig. 30). The Helex is a single Nitinol wire in a helical configuration which is covered by an expanded polytetrafluoroethylene patch. Pathologists will encounter these devices in explanted hearts on the surgical bench as well as in the autopsy suite.

Pathology of Closure Devices

Several types of complications have been reported for closure devices. The most straightforward is the failure to fully close the defect resulting in residual shunting. These devices work to close the defects at least in part via thrombosis with subsequent organization; if the thrombosis extends beyond the defect on the device, thromboemboli may result. Inadequate fixation of the device within the defect, or a device-defect size mismatch can result in device embolization. Fractures of various device components, air embolism at the time of device deployment, infection, device erosion through

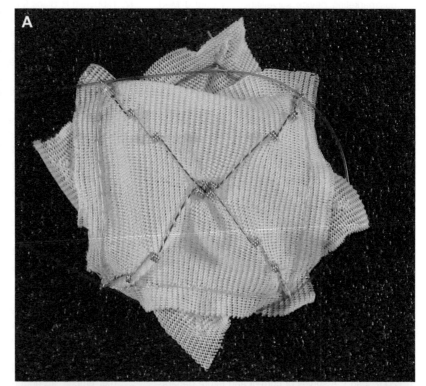

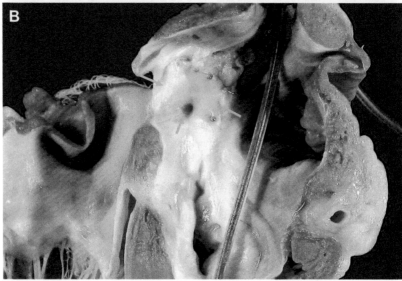

Fig. 30. STARFlex closure device. (*A*) Gross photograph of an undeployed device. (*B*) Gross photograph of the left atrial aspect of a STARFlex closure device (*arrows*) that has had excellent tissue ingrowth into the interstices of the Dacron occluder to the point where the device is indistinct.

adjacent tissues with perforation and development of new arrhythmias have also been reported. A number of devices are in development, with the trends being defect-specific design and minimization of the amount of foreign material left in the patient, including the use of biodegradable components.[46]

REFERENCES

1. Hauser RG. Here we go again - Another failure of postmarketing device surveillance. N Engl J Med 2012;366:873–5.

2. Resnic FS, Normand ST. Postmarketing surveillance of medical devices - filling in the gaps. N Engl J Med 2012;366:875–7.

3. Kuehn BM. Advocates call for FDA to take tougher stance on postmarket safety studies. JAMA 2011; 306:1639–42.

4. Padera RF, Schoen FJ. Cardiovascular applications of biomaterials. In: Ratner B, Hoffman A, Schoen FJ, et al, editors. Biomaterials science: an introduction to materials in medicine. 2nd edition. San Diego (CA): Elsevier Science; 2004. p. 470–94.

5. Serruys PW, de Jaegere P, Kiemeneij F, et al. A comparison of balloon-expandable-stent implantation with balloon angioplasty in patients with coronary artery disease. N Engl J Med 1994;331:489–95.

6. Agostoni P, Valgimigli M, Biondi-Zoccai GG, et al. Clinical effectiveness of bare-metal stenting compared with balloon angioplasty in total coronary occlusions: insights from a systematic overview of randomized trials in light of the drug-eluting stent era. Am Heart J 2006;151(3):682–9.

7. Serruys PW, Kutryk MJ, Ong AT. Coronary artery stents. N Engl J Med 2006;354:483–95.

8. Daemen J, Serruys PW. Drug-eluting stent update 2007: part I. A survey of current and future generation drug-eluting stents: meaningful advances or more of the same? Circulation 2007;116:316–28.

9. Daemen J, Serruys PW. Drug-eluting stent update 2007: part II: unsettled issues. Circulation 2007; 116:961–8.

10. Poon M, Badimon JJ, Fuster V. Overcoming restenosis with sirolimus: from alphabet soup to clinical reality. Lancet 2002;359:619–22.

11. Nakazawa G, Finn AV, Kolodgie FD, et al. A review of current devices and a look at new technology: drug eluting stents. Expert Rev Med Devices 2009;6:33–42.

12. Ramcharitar S, Serruys PW. Fully biodegradable coronary stents: progress to date. Am J Cardiovasc Drugs 2008;8:305–14.

13. Waksman R, Pakala R. Biodegradable and bioabsorbable stents. Curr Pharm Des 2010;16:4041–51.

14. Pedon L, Zennaro M, Calzolari D, et al. Strut fracture: a further concern with drug-eluting stents. J Cardiovasc Med (Hagerstown) 2008;9(9):949–52.

15. Stone JR, Basso C, Baandrup UT, et al. Recommendations for processing cardiovascular surgical pathology specimens: a consensus statement from the Standards and Definitions Committee of the Society of Cardiovascular Pathology and the Association for European Cardiovascular Pathology. Cardiovasc Pathol 2012;21:2–16.

16. Burke A, Tavora F. Coronary stents. In: Burke A, Tavora F, editors. Practical cardiovascular pathology. Philadelphia: Lippincott Williams & Wilkins; 2011. p. 104–8.

17. Rippstein P, Black MK, Boivin M, et al. Comparison of processing and sectioning methodologies for arteries containing metallic stents. J Histochem Cytochem 2006;54:673–81.

18. Kumar AH, McCauley SD, Hynes BG, et al. Improved protocol for processing stented porcine coronary arteries for immunostaining. J Mol Histol 2011;42:187–93.

19. Bradshaw SH, Kennedy L, Dexter DF, et al. A practical method to rapidly dissolve metallic stents. Cardiovasc Pathol 2009;18:127–33.

20. Nakazawa G. Stent thrombosis of drug eluting stent: pathological perspective. J Cardiol 2011;58:84–91.

21. Vorpahl M, Yazdani SK, Nakano M, et al. Pathobiology of stent thrombosis after drug-eluting stent implantation. Curr Pharm Des 2010;16:4064–71.

22. Finn AV, Nakazawa G, Joner M, et al. Vascular responses to drug eluting stents: importance of delayed healing. Arterioscler Thromb Vasc Biol 2007; 27:1500–10.

23. Virmani R, Farb A. Pathology of in-stent restenosis. Curr Opin Lipidol 1999;10:499–506.

24. Welt FG, Rogers C. Inflammation and restenosis in the stent era. Arterioscler Thromb Vasc Biol 2002; 22:1769–76.

25. Mehta RI, Solis OE, Jahan R, et al. Hydrophilic polymer emboli: an under-recognized iatrogenic cause of ischemia and infarct. Mod Pathol 2010;23:921–30.

26. Baughman KL, Jarcho JA. Bridge to life – cardiac mechanical support. N Engl J Med 2007;357:846–9.

27. Miller LW, Pagani FD, Russell SD, et al. Use of a continuous-flow device in patients awaiting heart transplantation. N Engl J Med 2007;357:885–96.

28. Slaughter MS, Rogers JG, Milano CA, et al. Advanced heart failure treated with continuous-flow left ventricular assist device. N Engl J Med 2009; 361:2241–51.

29. Fang JC. Rise of the machines - left ventricular assist devices as permanent therapy for advanced heart failure. N Engl J Med 2009;361:2282–5.

30. Birks EJ. Myocardial recovery in patients with chronic heart failure: is it real? J Card Surg 2010; 25:472–7.

31. Krishnamani R, DeNofrio D, Konstam MA. Emerging ventricular assist devices for long-term cardiac support. Nat Rev Cardiol 2010;7:71–6.

32. De Sousa CF, Brito FD, de Lima VC, et al. Percutaneous mechanical assistance for the failing heart. J Interven Cardiol 2010;23:195–202.

33. Lee MS, Makkar RR. Percutaneous left ventricular support devices. Cardiol Clin 2006;24:265–75.

34. Roussel JC, Senage T, Baron O, et al. CardioWest total artificial heart: a single-center experience with 42 patients. Ann Thorac Surg 2009;87:124–9.

35. Padera RF. Pathology of cardiac assist devices. In: McManus BM, Braunwald E, editors. Atlas of cardiovascular pathology for the clinician. 2nd edition. Philadelphia: Current Medicine; 2008. p. 257–73.

36. Padera RF. Infection in ventricular assist devices: the role of biofilm. Cardiovasc Pathol 2006;15: 264–70.

37. Hannan MM, Husain S, Mattner F, et al. Working formulation for the standardization of definitions of infections in patients using ventricular assist devices. J Heart Lung Transplant 2011;30:375–84.

38. Mudd JO, Cuda JD, Halushka M, et al. Fusion of aortic valve commissures in patients supported by a continuous axial flow left ventricular assist device. J Heart Lung Transplant 2008;27:1269–74.

39. Atlee JL, Bernstein AD. Cardiac rhythm management devices (part I): indications, device selection, and function. Anesthesiology 2001;95:1265–80.

40. Kusumoto FM, Goldschlager N. Device therapy for cardiac arrhythmias. JAMA 2002;287:1848–52.

41. Haqqani HM, Mond HG. The implantable cardioverter-defibrillator lead: principles, progress and promises. Pacing Clin Electrophysiol 2009;32:1336–53.

42. Amin MS, Ellenbogen KA. The effect of device advisories on implantable cardioverter-defibrillator therapy. Curr Cardiol Rep 2010;12:361–6.

43. Uslan DZ. Infections of electrophysiologic cardiac devices. Expert Rev Med Devices 2008;5:183–95.

44. Baddour LM, Epstein AE, Erickson CC, et al. Update on cardiovascular implantable electronic device infections and their management: a scientific statement from the American Heart Association. Circulation 2010;121:458–77.

45. Kim MS, Klein AJ, Carroll JD. Transcatheter closure of intracardiac defects in adults. J Interven Cardiol 2007;20:524–45.

46. Majunke N, Sievert H. ASD/PFO devices: what is in the pipeline? J Interven Cardiol 2007;20:517–23.

Index

Note: Page numbers of article titles are in **boldface** type.

A

Abdominal aortic aneurysm
   histologic findings in, 429
   incidence of, 428
Allograft failure
   acute rejection, 495
   coronary artery disease in, 494–495
Amputation specimen, vascular disease in, 450–451
Amyloidosis
   differential diagnosis of, 402
   H&E staining in, 401–403
   on native heart biopsy, 401–405
   prognosis in, 404–405
   subtyping of, 402–403
      techniques in, 403–404
   types of amyloid involving heart, 402
Aneurysmal disease
   ascending aortic, 421, 424–428
   familial thoracic, 426
   in medium-sized arteries, 435–436
      degenerative changes, acquired, 436
      fibromuscular dysplasia in, 436–437
      gross assessment of, 436
      hypertensive changes, 436
      microscopic features in, 436
      microvascular, 436, 438
      Mönckeberg's calcification, 438
      mycotic aneurysm, 438
      secondary to infection, 436, 438
      secondary to inflammatory degeneration, 436
Angiosarcoma, 478–479
   differential diagnosis of, 479
   hemangioma and lymphangioma *vs.,* 473
Aorta
   abdominal aortic aneurysm of, 428–429
   aneurysm types in
      diffuse, 419–420
      fusiform, 419–420
      imaging of, 420
      saccular, 419–421
   aortitis of
      from IgG4-related systemic disease, 428–429
      histopathologic classification scheme for, 428–432
      non-syphilitic infectious, 428
      syphilitic, 427–428
   ascending aneurysms
      genetic disease causes of, 421, 424–426
      non-genetic disease cause of, 426–428

   congenital abnormalities of, 430
   fibroinflammatory disease of, 431–432
   giant cell arteritis of, 427
   gross features of
      atherosclerotic plaques, 418
      color, 418
      tree barking, 418
   grossing considerations for, 417–418
      histology, 417–418
      orientation of tissue, 417–418
   microscopic features of
      diffuse medial degeneration, 421, 424
      elastic fiber fragmentation, 421, 424
      inflammation, 421–423
      laminar medial necrosis, 421, 423
      medial degeneration, 421–423
   pathology of, **417–433**
   surgical
      congenital abnormalities in, 430
      fibroinflammatory disease in, 431–432
      tumors in, 430–431
      unusual findings in, 430–432
   Takayasu arteritis of, 427
   tumors in, 430–431
Aortic valve. See also *Native Cardiac Valve pathology.*
   anatomy of, 328–329
   bicuspid, aneurysm in, 416
   regurgitant, 332
      aortic diseases and, 332–333
      aortic root disorders and, 333
      congenitally bicuspid valve and, 332
      cusps in, 333–334
      infective endocarditis and, 332
      post-inflammatory-rheumatic valves and, 331–332
   stenotic of, 329
      congenitally bicuspid, 330
      congenitally unicuspid, 330–331
      degenerative calcific, 329–330
      post-inflammatory-rheumatic, 330, 332
Aortitis
   from IgG4-related systemic disease, 428
   giant cell, 422–423
   histopathologic classification of, 428
   lymphoplasmacytic, 422–423
   non-syphilitic infectious, 428
   syphilitic, 427–428
Arterial tortuosity syndrome, 426
Atherosclerosis, 447–448

Surgical Pathology 5 (2012) 523–528
doi:10.1016/S1875-9181(12)00072-4

Atherosclerosis (*continued*)
  in thrombectomy, embolectomy, and
    endarterectomy specimens, 448, 450
  lipid accumulation in, 447–448
Atrial septal defects, occlusion devices for. See
  Occlusion device(s).

B

Behçet's disease, 443, 445–447
Bicuspid aortic valve and aneurysm (BAV), 426
Biopsies
  of cardiac transplants, **371–400** (*See* Cardiac
    transplant biopsies)
  of native heart, **401–416** (*See* Native heart
    biopsies)
Blood cyst, hemangioma and lymphangioma *vs.,*
  473
Buerger's disease (thromboangiitis obliterans), 443,
  445–446

C

Carcinoid valve disease, tricuspid valve regurgitation
  in, 343–345
Cardiac explant
  allograft
    coronary artery disease in, 495
    failed, 494
  coronary artery dissection of, 486–488
  diagnosis of, 492
  dissection of
    for cardiomyopathy, 492–493
    for ischemic heart disease, 485–491
    four chamber long axis cut in, 492–493
  examination of, **485–495**
  histology of, 491
  transplant procedure, 485
  ventricular examination of
    cross-section approach to, 486, 489
    left side dissection, 488–491
    right side dissection, 486, 488, 490–491
    shape of septum in, 489, 491
  with congenital heart disease, 492
  with valvular disease, 492
Cardiac transplant biopsies, **371–400**
  allograft coronary disease on, 389–390
  communcation of results of, 398
  findings in biopsy site, 382, 385
  for acute cellular rejection
    grading for, 373–378
    indications for therapeutic intervention in, 378
    morphology of, 373
  for antibody-mediated rejection
    immunostaining in, 378, 380
    indications for therapeutic intervention in, 381
    morphology of, 378–379

  infection in
    Chagas disease, 386–388
    cytomegalovirus, 386–387
    fungal, 388
    Toxoplasma gondii, 386–387
  International Society for Heart and Lung
    Transplantation 2004 and 2011 grading
    system for, 376–378
  microinfarcts on, 389–390
  other findings
    primary disease recurrence in allograft,
      381–382
  peritransplant ischemic injury in
    early, 382–383
    healing phase, 383–384
    vs. acute cellular rejection, 382, 384
  post-transplant lymphoproliferative disorder,
    389–390
  processing of, 371–372
  prognosis for transplant recipients, 398
  protocols for, 372
  quilty effect in, 385–386
  requirements for, 371
  signout form for reporting results, 397
  specimen adequacy for, 371–372
  subendocardial myocyte vacuolization on,
    389–390
  tissue artifacts on
    contraction bands, 393
    edema, true interstitial, 391
    fat/mesothelial cells, 395
    foreign body, 396
    hemorrhage, 392
    intravascular lymphocytes, 394
    other than myocardium, 396
    telescoping (intusssuception), 393
    thrombus, 392
Cardiac tumor(s), **453–483**
  anatomic distribution of, 454
  ball-valve effect of, 453, 455
  benign primary
    cystic tumor of atrioventriciular node,
      475–476
    fibroma, 468–470
    hamartoma of mature cardiac myocytes,
      470–471
    hemangioma, 471–473
    lipomatous hypertrophy of interatrial septum,
      473–475
    lymphangioma, 471–473
    myxoma, 456–461
    papillary fibroelastoma, 461–465
    paraganglioma, 476–478
    rhabdomyoma, 465–467
  frequency of, by age and tumor type, 454
  malignant primary
    angiosarcoma, 477–479

lymphoma, 480–482
    undifferentiated pleomorphic sarcoma,
        479–480
    pericardial involvement of, 453–455
    syndromes associated with, 456
Cardiovascular medical device(s)
    coronary artery stents, 498–503
    pathologic evaluation of, **497–521**
    reactions to, 497–498
    risks with, 497
    ventricular assist devices, 504–517
Chagas disease, in cardiac transplant biopsy,
    386–388
Churg-Strauss syndrome, 442, 445–446
Congenital heart disease, in cardiac explant, 492
Coronary artery, in cardiac explant, dissection of,
    486–488
Coronary artery disease, in allograft failure, 494–495
Coronary artery stents
    bare metal, 498, 501
    classification of, 498
    drug-eluting, 498, 501–502
    embolic material distal to, 502–503
    gross evaluation of
        dissection and radiography for, 498–499
        sectioning of non-stented artery portions,
            499–500
    intimal proliferation with, 500, 502
    microscopic evaluation of, specialized labs for,
        500
    processing of stented segment of artery,
        498–500
    restenosis with, 500–502
    thrombosis with, 500–501
Cystic tumor of atrioventricular node, 473, 475–476

E

Ebstein's anomaly, tricuspid valve regurgitation in,
    343
Ehlers-Danlos syndrome, ascending aortic aneurysm
    in, 425
Embolus, septic, 448, 450
Epithelioid hemagngioendothelioma, angiosarcoma
    vs., 479

F

Fibroma
    differential diagnosis of, 470
    gross features of, 468
    hamartoma of mature cardiac myocytes vs., 471
    microscopic features of, 468–469
    pattern recognition in, 469
Fibrosarcoma, undifferentiated pleomorphic
    sarcoma vs., 480
Fungal endocarditis, active, 349

G

Giant cell arteritis (GCA)
    gross assessment of, 439
    "healed arteritis," 440–441
    microscopic features of
        chronic inflammation, 439–440
        intimal hyperplasia, 440
        lymphohistiocytic infiltrate to internal elastic
            lamina, 439–440
    prognosis for, 440
    temporal artery in normal aging and, 440, 442
    thoracic artery aneurysm in, 427
Giant cell myocarditis, 406–407, 409
    sarcoidosis vs., 410
Glycogen storage disorders, on native heart biopsy,
    411–413
Granular cell tumor
    paraganglioma vs., 478
    rhabdomyoma vs., 467

H

Hamartoma of mature cardiac myocytes (HMCH),
    470–471
    differential diagnosis of, 471
    fibroma vs., 470
Hemangioma, 471–473
Histiocytic cardiomyopathy, rhabdomyoma vs.,
    467
Hypersensitivitiy myocarditis, 406–407, 409
    sarcoidosis vs., 410
Hypertrophic cardiomyopathy, hamartoma of mature
    cardiac myocytes vs., 471

I

Infection, in cardiac transplant biopsy, 386–387
Infective endocarditis
    active
        gross pathology of, 347–349
        vegetations in, 347
    acute, 347
    chronic, 347
        pathologoy of, 349
    healing, 348
    in pulmonic and tricuspid valves, 345–347
    prosthetic valve-associated, 357, 360–361
Inflammatory myofibroblastic humor, fibroma vs.,
    469–470
International Society for Heart and Lung
    Transplantation 2004 and 2011 grading system for
    cardiac transplant biopsies, 376–378
Iron overload, on native heart biopsy, 410–412

K

Kaposi sarcoma, angiosarcoma vs., 479

L

Lambls' excrescence, myxoma *vs.*, 461, 465
Leukocytoclastic vasculitis, 442, 444–446
Lipomatous hypertrophy of interatrial septum, 473–475
Loeys-Dietz syndrome, ascending aortic aneurysm in, 425–426
Lymphangioma, 471–473
Lymphocytic myocarditis, 406–407, 409
  sarcoidosis *vs.*, 410
Lymphoma
  differential diagnosis of, 473, 480
  gross features of, 480–481
  microscopic features of, 480, 482
Lymphoproliferative disorder, post-transplant, 389–390
Lysosomal storage disorders, on native heart biopsy, 413–414

M

Marfan syndrome, ascending aortic aneurysm in, 425
Mesothelioma, angiosarcoma *vs.*, 479
Mitral valve
  anatomy of, 334
  insufficiency of, from regurgitation, 335, 337–342
  regurgitant
    chordal causes of, 340
    degenerative, 337
    drug-related, 339–340
    infective endocarditis and, 337, 339–340
    leaflet causes of, 335, 337–340
    mitral annular calcification, 341
    myxomatous valve disease and, 335, 337–338
    papillary muscle dysfunction and, 341–342
    ventricular causes of, 340–341
  stenotic, rheumatic, 334–336
Mönckeberg's calcification, 447
Myocarditis
  acute necrotizing eosinophilic, 408–409
  giant cell, 406–407, 409
  hypersensitivity, 406–407, 409
  immunohistochemistry for, 409
  lymphocytic, 406–407, 409
  molecular analyses for, 409
  on native biopsy
    histologic subtypes of, 406
    idiopathic or secondary, 405
    microscopic features of, 406–407, 409
    presentation of, 405–406
Myxoma
  differential diagnosis of, 459, 461
  gross features of, 456–457
  microscopic features of, 456, 458–460
Myxosarcoma, undifferentiated pleomorphic sarcoma *vs.*, 480–481

N

Native cardiac valve pathology, **327–352.** See also named valve, e.g., *Aortic valve.*
  conclusions on evaluation of, 349
  evaluation for
    gross examination in, 327–328
    sectioning in, 328
    stains in, 328
    ultrastructural, 328
  of aortic valve, 329–334
  of mitral valve, 334–342
  of pulmonary valve, 342–348
  of tricuspid valve, 342–348
Native heart biopsies
  cardiac amyloidosis on, 401–402
  conditions with diagnostic features on, 401
  glycogen storage disorders on, 411–413
  iron overload on, 410–412
  lysosomnal storage disorders on, 413–414
  myocarditis on, 405–409
  sarcoidosis on, 409–410
  stains for, 401

O

Occlusion device(s)
  Amplatzer device, 518
  for atrial and ventricular septal defects, 517–519
  Helex, 519
  pathology of
    component fracture, 519
    erosion through adjacent tissues, 520
    failure to close, 519
    thrombosis, 519
  StarFLEX device, 518–519

P

Pacemakers and implantable cardioverter-defibrillators
  described, 509–510
  patholgist evaluation of, 511
  pathology of
    battery depletion, 513
    biomaterial interaction with host tissue, 514
    device failure, 513
    fibrous reaction to electrode tip, 516
    lead-related, 514–515
    thrombosis of leads, 516
Papillary fibroelastoma (PFE)
  differential diagnosis of, 461
  gross features of, 461–463
  microscopic features of, 464
  myxoma *vs.*, 459
  pattern recognition in, 464
  secondary, 463

Paraganglioma
    gross appearance of, 476–478
    microscopic appearance of, 477–478
Polyarteritis nodosa, 442, 444, 446
Prosthetic heart valve(s)
    autograft, 365
    bioprosthetic, 353–354, 356–360
        calcification and valvular stenosis of,
            362–363
        Carpenter-Edwards bovine pericardial,
            361–363
        Hancock porcine, 359, 363
        Medtronic Freestyle stentless porcine, 360
        Sorin Mitroflow, 358
        St. Jude bicor, 360
        St. Jude bileaflet tilting disc, 360
    complications of, 360–363
        calcification, 360, 362–363
        fungal infection, 360
        infective endocarditis, 357, 360
        non-structural, 362–364
        pannus overgrowth with regurgitation or
            stenosis, 363–364
        paravalvular leaks, 362
        structural, 362–363
        structural/mechanical, 360–363
        thromboembolic, 357
    evaluation of, **353–369**
    failure of, causes of, 354
    homograft, 364–365
    in development, 366
    mechanical, 353–354
        bileaflet tilting-disc, 356–357
        Harken caged disc, 356
        Medtronic-Hall single leaflet tilting disc, 356
        Starr-Edwards caged ball, 356
        types of, 355–357
    pathologic features of, assessment of, 354
    transcatheter aortic valve implantation, 365–366
Pulmonary valve(s)
    anatomy of, 342–343
    bicuspid, regurgitant and stenotic, 345
    infective endocarditis in, 345–348
    regurgitatant, carcinoid valve disease and,
        343–345
    unicuspid, stenotic, 345

R

Rhabdomyoma
    differential diagnosis of, 467
    fibroma vs., 470
    gross features of, 465–466
    hamartoma of mature cardiac myocytes vs.,
        471
    microscopic features of, 465–466
    pattern recognition in, 465

S

Sarcoidosis
    differential diagnosis of, 410
    fibrosis in, 409–410
    granulomatous inflammation in, 409–410
    on native heart biopsy, 409–410
Sarcoma
    hamartoma of mature cardiac myocytes vs., 471
    undifferentiated pleomorphic, 479–480
    with myxoid features, myxoma vs., 459
Shunt revision specimen, vascular disease in, 451
Small vessel vasculitide(s)
    antineutrophil-associated cytoplasmic antibodies
        in, 442, 444–445
    Behçet's disease, 443, 445–447
    Buerger's disease (thromboangiitis obliterans),
        443, 445–446
    Churg-Strauss syndrome, 442, 445–446
    features of common, 446
    leukocytoclastic vasculitis, 442, 444–446
    microscopic features of, 443–447
    polyarteritis nodosa, 442, 444, 446
    Wegener's granulomatosis, 442–443, 446
Stenosis
    of aortic valve, 330–332
    of mitral valve, 334–336
    of pulmonary valve, 345

T

Takayasu arteritis, aortic, 427
Temporal arteritis. See Giant cell arteritis (GCA
    [Temporal arteritis]).
Thrombosis(es)
    in thrombectomy, embolectomy, and
        endarterectomy specimens, 448–450
    of coronary artery stents, 500–501
    of occlusion devices, 519
    of pacemaker and impantable cardioverter-
        defibrillator leads, 516
    of ventricular assist devices, 509, 511–513
Tricuspid valve
    anatomy of, 342
    infective endocarditis in, 345–347
    regurgitant
        carcinoid valve disease and, 343–345
        Ebstein's anomaly and, 343
        flail leaflet and, 343
        rheumatic involvement in, 343
Turner syndrome, ascending aortic aneurysm in,
    426

V

Valve(s)
    aortic, 328–334, 426
    mitral, 334–342

Valve(s) (*continued*)
  native, **327–352**
  prosthetic, **353–369**
  pulmonary, 342–348
Vascular graft/conduit specimen, vascular disease in, 451
Vasculitis. See *Small vessel vasculitide(s).*
Vein stripping/thromboplebitis specimen, vascular disease in, 451
Ventricular assist device(s) (VADs), 504–506
  CardiacAssist Tandem Heart, 505
  gross evaluation of
    left ventricular, 506–507
    right ventricular, 507–508
  pathology of, 507, 509
    cuspal fusion, 509, 513
    impingement on intraventricular septum, 509, 515
    infection, 509–510
    outflow anastomotic thrombosis, 509, 513
    thrombi within heart, 509, 514
    thrombosis, 509, 511–512
  Syncardia Total Artificial Hart, 506

Thoratec HeartMate II, 505, 507
Thoratec HeartMate PVAD, 505
Thoratec HeartMate XVE, 504
Thoratec IVAD, 505
Ventricular septal defets, occlusion devices for. *See* Occlusion device(s)
Vessels
  aneurysmal disease of, 435–439
  atherosclerosis in, 447–448
  giant cell arteritis in, 439–442, 446
  small, vasculitis in, 442–447
  surgical pathology of, **435–451**
    general considerations, 435
    in amputations, 450–451
    in embolectomy, endarterectomy, and thrombectomy specimens, 448–450
    in shunt revisions, 451
    in vascular grafts/conduits, 451
    in vein stripping/thrombophlebitis, 451

W

Wegener's granulomatosis, 442–443, 446

Moving?

Make sure your subscription moves with you!

To notify us of your new address, find your **Clinics Account Number** (located on your mailing label above your name), and contact customer service at:

Email: journalscustomerservice-usa@elsevier.com

800-654-2452 (subscribers in the U.S. & Canada)
314-447-8871 (subscribers outside of the U.S. & Canada)

Fax number: 314-447-8029

Elsevier Health Sciences Division
Subscription Customer Service
3251 Riverport Lane
Maryland Heights, MO 63043

*To ensure uninterrupted delivery of your subscription, please notify us at least 4 weeks in advance of move.

ELSEVIER

Printed and bound by CPI Group (UK) Ltd, Croydon, CR0 4YY

03/10/2024

01040351-0001